JAN 1 8 2016

9-29-16(2)

EMBRACING A.D.D.

EMBRACING A.D.D.

A Healing Perspective

Lynn Weiss, PhD

TAYLOR TRADE PUBLISHING

Lanham • Boulder • New York • London

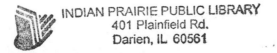

Published by Taylor Trade Publishing
An imprint of The Rowman & Littlefield Publishing Group, Inc.
4501 Forbes Boulevard, Suite 200, Lanham, Maryland 20706
www.rowman.com

Unit A, Whitacre Mews, 26-34 Stannary Street, London SE11 4AB

Distributed by NATIONAL BOOK NETWORK

British Library Cataloguing in Publication Information Available

Library of Congress Cataloging-in-Publication Data
Weiss, Lynn.
  Embracing A.D.D. : a healing perspective / Lynn Weiss Ph.D.
    pages cm
  ISBN 978-1-58979-837-3 (pbk. : alk. paper) — ISBN 978-1-58979-838-0
(electronic) 1. Attention-deficit disorder in adults—Popular works. 2. Attention-
deficit disorder in adults—Treatment—Popular works. 3. Self-care, Health.
I. Title.
  RC394.A85W446 2015
  616.85'89—dc23

                                                                    2015006760

∞™ The paper used in this publication meets the minimum requirements of
American National Standard for Information Sciences—Permanence of Paper
for Printed Library Materials, ANSI/NISO Z39.48-1992.

Printed in the United States of America

CONTENTS

PREFACE

I'm a social scientist and field researcher whose strongest skill is my ability to use observation to learn, in contrast to learning about things taught by others. First I sense things, and only later follow what I suspect with questioning, further observation, and historical review.

Experiencing how and why something functions the way it does is more useful to me than learning what something is called or memorizing how something works. I want to know the effects of the environment and my involvement in what I am studying before I accept the results of anyone else's study.

In this book, I'm going to tell you many stories of people who are endowed with a brain construction labeled Attention Deficit Disorder (ADD) or Attention Deficit Hyperactivity Disorder (ADHD). (For purposes of this book, we'll call them both ADD.) You'll be mentored, not just by me, but by the people who share their experiences in the telling of their stories. Finally, you will be provided with a paradigm for experiencing ADD that is different from the medically identified definition with which many of you may be familiar—one that embraces the value of diversity within each of us.

My perspective has come from firsthand observations rather than from textbooks or "experts" or from anyone with a predominantly Linear brainstyle. Though I know the more popular belief about ADD—as is identified within the *Diagnostic and Statistical Manual of Mental Disorders*, published by the American Psychiatric Association—I have increasingly shifted away from the medical model in which it is framed.

I am by no means the first to consider a nonmedical approach. Others who laid the groundwork for looking at ADD from a different perspective than the medical model include James J. Chriss, associate professor of sociology at Cleveland State University, who wrote in 1937: "The cure (for ADD) preceded the ailment. Before the disorder was named, drug treatment had been developed to subdue children's unruly behavior." (*Social Control: An Introduction*, Cambridge, CB 1HR UK, and Malden MA 02148, USA: Polity Press, 2013.)

Thomas Szasz reiterated in his book *Pharmacracy: Medicine and Politics in America* in 2001 (Westport, CT: Praeger), "Mental diseases are invented and then given a name, for example attention deficit hyperactivity disorder (ADHD)."

Jerome C. Wakefield, 2002, considered ADD to be a normal response "to the constrictions of normal childhood activity" in "Values and the Validity of Diagnostic Criteria: Disvalued versus Disordered Conditions of Childhood and Adolescence," pp. 148–64, in *Descriptions and Prescriptions: Values, Mental Disorders, and the DSMs*, ed. J. Z. Sadler. Baltimore: Johns Hopkins University Press.

One might wonder why there is such a discrepancy between the beliefs held by different professionals working with ADD. I've come to understand that frequently people experience situations and outcomes in dissimilar ways, coming away with differing conclusions that reflect their experience and the way in which their own perceptual system is constructed. I also know that the social structures and cultural settings in which each of us lives will affect our perceptions. So, too, will our personalities, brainstyles, and life experiences from childhood on impact what we experience.

There is little doubt in my mind that I see the perspective I do because of my brainstyle, which, by the way is very ADD, Analogue, and Nonlinear. What I choose to do in this book is to give you a perspective to consider, one some of you will find rewarding and freeing. Other readers may be uncomfortable with the direction I've taken. Perhaps there will be readers who discount my perspective altogether.

Remember how you view any suggestions. If what you read resonates with your thinking and feeling, "It feels right for me," then embrace it. If it does not feel comfortable or right for you, then set it aside as you shift toward a perspective with which you are comfortable.

I know that my perspective stems from an intense desire to see the best in people, to honor what each of us has rather than judge or dishonor what we don't have. I am not the better because I can view another as lesser. I experience our differences as simply different. I believe that there is a place for every one of us in the big scheme of things.

As you read through this book, I want you to notice how you feel about what you read. Is it enlightening? Does it engender hope? Does the information give you something that you can make use of? Can you identify with what you are reading for yourself or someone you care about? What I ask you to do is make up your own mind about whether my perspective of ADD resonates for you or not.

I am about to bring you a perspective of ADD that belies the title given to this particular style of brain construction. I bring you a way of looking at yourself and your wonderful brainstyle not as a pathological phenomenon requiring repair, but as a valid, though different, way of thinking, behaving, and expressing all that you are.

From my professional observations and intimate involvement with ADD adults for the past twenty-five years, I have pursued a path I didn't expect to find, much less follow. I did not start out with a hypothesis or expectations of what I would discover.

I was initially introduced to the subject in the late 1970s when I was consulting in educational settings, preschool through primary grades. From time to time, children were being identified with ADD. At the time, this was not my specialty, so I primarily observed their behavior and found them to be active, yes, but not extraordinarily out-of-control. They were too young to stand out that much from their kinesthetic learning peers and too young to "diagnose" with certainty. By early 1980, I began to be exposed to ADD in teens and adults. The result was my massive involvement with ADD in adults from that time on.

Embracing ADD is the result of forty years of self-study, teaching, training, and consulting in the fields of learning differences, counseling, and psychotherapy. I conducted multiple interviews in which I was able to observe and dialogue with the many people who sought assistance with something they didn't understand. I started a program for individuals who thought they recognized ADD attributes in their thinking and behavior and chose to develop support groups from the very beginning of the adult movement.

Your job is to take from this book what works for you and set the rest aside. I trust you because, ultimately, you know more about yourself, what *fits* you, and what you need than I or anyone else ever could know. At least you will experience a sense of what is right for you and what isn't as you draw toward embracing what you are hearing, seeing, or experiencing. Trust yourself!

At this point, you may wish to use the simple Assessment Checklist in chapter 1 to ascertain a likelihood that you may have more attributes of Analogue brain processing (as people with an

ADD brainstyle have) than Linear brainstyle processing. If it turns out that you do lean in the ADD direction, you will likely benefit from discovering aspects of your *True You*. And when you ascertain your balance of ADD and Linear traits, you can learn to heal the wounding that happened because of living and learning in a Linear culture, and determine how to prevent further damage from occurring.

You may also go directly to chapter 1 to discover the beginning of your journey to viewing ADD as a diversity issue. You may already know the balance of your brainstyle or you may wish to discover it later or never. The choice is up to you. And I trust you to know what feels right to you.

EMBRACING ACKNOWLEDGMENTS

Acknowledgments reflect the life-blood of any work; nowhere else is it more apparent than in the craft of writing. For, through this means of expression, a creation of the heart and mind, many perspectives, skills, and talents are required. More than ever before do I realize the limitations of my own input to the completed manuscript. And so, I wish to say thank you to the many contributors to this book.

All my gratitude began when I was in school, from kindergarten on—I say thank you to the many teachers good and bad, inspirational and hurtful, and, most of all, visionary, as they saw and guided the skills and talents that I, the student, possessed.

Most important to this book are the many people who talked to me in past years—you told me me your stories and opened yourselves to share your pains and wishes, needs and healings. Thank you to each and every one who contributed from your heart and soul. You know who you are. I know you.

Next are those whose specific jobs and interests shaped the tangible outcome of the ADD story with its transition to more than it was originally.

John Rubel, Psy D., who has stayed with me through my series of ADD books, bringing a Linear perspective to my far-reaching Analog vision, affirming and reaching to understand a mind so different from his own. Together, the best of our diverse learning styles have touched the understanding reflected in this book.

And thank you, Janis Dworkis, my initial writing teacher for my first ADD manuscript in the early nineties and a current editor who doctored this manuscript for initial submission to Taylor Trade Publishing. Thank you Janis, friend and editor.

And finally, I wish to acknowledge Taylor Trade Publishing for standing by my side through the many years of ADD development from "ADD, a Disorder" to the metamorphosis to "ADD, a Diversity Issue."

Thank you to editorial director Rick Rinehart, associate marketing manager Kalen Landow, publicity manager Sharon Kunz, assistant editor Karie Simpson, and production editor Alden Perkins, as well as to the many who make up Taylor's support staff. You are one mighty team, who feels more like a family than the Big Company in the sky.

Your grateful author,
Lynn Weiss, PhD
2015

1

DIVERSITY, NOT DISORDER

The year was 1986 when I was counseling a family with an ADD son. The family had come in periodically to update their work with their son's school and try to integrate social training he was receiving elsewhere as he moved into adolescence. Rick was a well-behaved, outgoing young man who was learning to fit into the school learning system, though at times it was hard.

In those days, the common belief in the professional world was that ADD disappeared at puberty. But it seemed to the parents that the stresses of maneuvering through ever-more-complicated settings in middle school were becoming overwhelming, primarily because of the organizational skills and interactive requirements of the social scene with peers, teachers, and administrators.

The family decided to launch a two-pronged approach to curb the stresses Rick was facing. He was placed on a trial dosage of Ritalin simultaneously to being referred to a small group of similarly challenged young adolescents facing interpersonal and mildly disruptive social and communicational behaviors. The group's licensed counselor was a young adult with an ADD brainstyle who could empathize with the students while helping them develop and maintain appropriate limits. He also served as a role model for success.

By the end of the year, Rick was able to discontinue his meds, having had time to practice the skills he needed to succeed throughout the rest of high school.

I began to think about my experience with this family and became aware of other adolescents and young adults who were struggling in high school and later with attempts to continue their education in local community colleges. ADD appeared to surface as a probable culprit.

One day, I mused on my talk-radio show that it appeared that ADD did not go anywhere at puberty, as was commonly believed by medical practitioners, and was in all probability something with which a person is born and carries throughout life, for better or worse.

Well, I'm here to tell you, the talk lines lit up, suddenly blinking wildly with people seeking information about what I had said about ADD in adulthood. Word was passed to me that the station's switchboard was becoming overloaded with calls from people waiting to talk to me about ADD. Nothing like this had happened before. Here was a situation that was extending beyond the time I had on air. What was I to do? Little did I know that the marathon had begun, to end I knew not where. And two decades later, it's still moving along!

A meeting with the station management proved a success when I asked if they would sponsor a public gathering for people with an interest in adult ADD. Within ten days, with the help of two local college educators, I held a ninety-minute informal meeting for adults who were interested in ADD on the job, in adult education, and in their relationships—a meeting that didn't break up for three hours. I have to say that the information available was scanty, but the enthusiasm and desire for assistance was strong.

Due to public interest, I started holding information groups at my clinic, and together, the participants and I began to figure out what was needed to help adults still needing to deal with ADD in themselves. We shared ideas, and information such as "This works for me," and "Oh, I heard about this . . ." A true grassroots support group began, and we all learned together. It was an exciting and heady time.

Meanwhile, I was doing assessments of people who thought they might be ADD and I discovered an inordinately high level of accurate self-diagnosis, a conclusion that twenty-six years later still holds true. People, and often their closest friends and family, recognize typical ADD attributes in a flash.

One day, a woman who loved to read asked me to recommend a book to give her more understanding of what ADD was about. I had already researched this issue and had to tell her that no book was available in the popular self-help, trade book market at that time. There were a few short articles in professional journals that were tentative in their observations, providing little help for adults in their living with an ADD brainstyle.

So, in my typical ADD way, though I didn't yet know that I, too, was blessed with the brainstyle that had invaded my professional life, a thought flew through my head, and the words poured out of my mouth as I said, "Well, I guess I'll have to write one." By the year 1992, *Attention Deficit Disorder in Adults*, first edition, was published. In no time, a second printing was required and the book became the first best seller on adult ADD in the US market.

Remember—all this time I was a radio talk-show host in a major market with lots of opportunities to network with other media outlets, in addition to having a publishing company that did a wonderful job of spreading the information to media opportunities across the country. The media responded with radio, television, and speaking opportunities flooding daily into my office. What fun as I made trips to New York City several times to do morning shows about this new phenomenon and welcomed the *CBS Evening News* to my office in Dallas. Speaking engagements took me coast-to-coast, and my as-yet-undiscovered ADD self discovered expressive skills I didn't know I had.

The gift of gab (what a wonderful ADD trait) that I used on the radio came in handy. And I recognized for the second time in my life that the minute a question was asked of me, I became instantly smart. I could speak what I didn't know I knew. Yet it came out with sparkling clarity, and I immediately knew that what I had said was true.

Only much later did I realize that all this time, I was using skills that I didn't realize were dependent upon my ADD brainstyle construction. Some insight came from my awareness of Howard Gardner's "Multiple Intelligences Theory," as you see I have strong intrapersonal and interpersonal intelligence skills. I didn't relate them for a long time to my interest and biases with ADD. A great deal more insight has gently emerged since the early days, thanks to my observational field work with ADD in adults.

As people told me their stories, I gained more and more information about the ADD brainstyle. You and every other person have a brainstyle—the unique manner in which you observe and receive information, and the way you associate, retain, recall, and express the information that you've received. As I worked with more and more people with an ADD brainstyle during those years, I obtained a perspective that did not follow the model I was originally trained to see. I began to notice firsthand what worked and what didn't with those who sought ADD counseling and assessment. Much like any teacher does as she puts in a couple years of hands-on work in a classroom after completing a formal education, I became increasingly clear about what people with an ADD brainstyle are like.

By then it was 1991 and 1992. A rewarding part of my contact with ADD audiences was the participants' gratitude for "being discovered" and understood. At that time, after saying it was my pleasure to be with them, I would laugh and quip, "I come as close to being ADD as you can be without really having it." Another year went by until I realized my shortsightedness. I realized without a doubt just how ADD I was and will always be.

I came to realize why I'd not seen my ADD before, caught as I was in the cultural party line that I *should* be able to do all the things that were impossibly hard for me to do. But it took until 1997 for me to be able to get my mind around what was happening to my self-image and to process through a very painful history of trying unbelievably hard but not achieving as I expected myself to achieve. Finally in 1997, I could write in an orderly way about my personal involvement.

MY PERSPECTIVE CHANGES

Throughout 1991 and 1992, I continued to see all kinds of people with all kinds of personalities and what turned out to be varying types of ADD. Thanks to my background in mental health counseling and psychotherapy, I could differentiate a mental health or addiction issue from ADD people whose behaviors and issues were situationally caused because of a lack of *fit* in relation to their ADD style of brain construction.

Initially, in the early 1990s, I heard words in casual conversation such as, "the booming, buzzing, confusion" of ADD. A family member might be spoken of more specifically. "He marches to his own drum." Sometimes it went as far as to say, "She's the black sheep in the family" or "I've never figured out what makes her tick."

Next, these grassroots observers talked about hearing phrases that a teacher or employer might use to describe the production and achievement results of a colleague, coworker, or student: "procrastinates, doesn't finish tasks, has a lot of unfulfilled potential, doesn't listen, is never still, goes like a whirlwind," or "never takes anything seriously."

Rarely were positive comments attributed to ADD. Instead, derogatory comments like "airhead," "space cadet," or "chatterbox" were said to describe people with ADD characteristics.

Qualitative judgments were made about motor activity, lack of impulse control, and poor organization and task completion.

Words from professionals were increasingly being touted, usually carrying a tone reflecting abnormality or a suggestion that something is wrong: attention-span deficiency, motor abnormality, emotional overreactivity to stress, excessive temper, hyperactivity, and, later, hypoactivity.

As a result of what I was hearing, I reviewed the current conversation about the ADD thinking of that time, much of which to date came from work with children. At first I accepted the medical model's perspective of ADD, passing on the idea that something is wrong or deficient about a person with ADD symptoms.

But, slowly, a discrepancy between the early thinking and languaging of ADD began to bother me. I didn't hear about any of the positive aspects of ADD. The descriptions voiced sounded more and more like arbitrary judgments. The result was a collision in my mind between the allopathic/medical model and my own growing sense that ADD is a brainstyle *difference*.

Increasingly, I became uneasy with the language of "suffering," of people with a "disorder." As a result, when the third edition of my book *Attention Deficit Disorder in Adults* was published, I changed the subtitle from, "Practical Help for Sufferers and Their Spouses," to "Practical Help and Understanding."

Thus, I "re-languaged" my original book, *Attention Deficit Disorder in Adults*, in its entirety so I wouldn't cringe when I read it or feel guilty when recommending it to someone to read.

I realized for the first time that ADD could be looked at from a sociocultural perspective that honored the diversification contributed by varying, but equally valued, types of brainstyles—brainstyles each of which fit some, but not all contexts. When I thought about trying to put a square peg in a round hole or getting a solid seat for a round peg placed in a square hole, I felt a familiar feeling—one I'd been feeling in relation to ADD.

Once I crossed this critical chasm of belief, I saw the importance of differences between the allopathic/medical model interpretations that deal with an illness/health model and a diversity model that I saw evolving.

Instead of only being uncomfortable with the terminology used in the ADD movement, I began to see as many wonderful attributes—no longer called symptoms—associated with ADD as difficulties. Examples of positive attributes of ADD included the ability to have visionary, expansive thought, to see the big picture, to be sensitive to patterns and relationships, and to recognize how things function. Often I saw creativity exuded with confidence and high energy expressed with flare and grace.

I also began to see how the channeling of ADD attributes into positive outlets that *fit* the parameters of the attributes was the key to a positive use of an ADD style of brain construction. I recall giving talks and saying, "You wouldn't send a fish to flying school, would you? They'd flunk wing training," after which the audience would howl with laughter and relief as the participants realized that maybe they weren't so impaired as they had come to believe.

DIVERSITY CONSIDERED

More and more I felt that the judgments about ADD, the disorder, were based on a unilateral belief system that was reflective of a Linear western sociocultural model—one in which a Linear style of perceiving, thinking about, and experiencing information and reaching goals was more valued than the Analogue style that reflected holistic, intuitive, functional ways of viewing information or achieving goals.

Particularly impacted were the institutions of education and medicine, both of which tended to reflect a monolithic perspective of what is considered the "right" and "wrong" ways to think and perform. Those people who functioned in this Linear style were frequently considered to be learning in the "right" way. They were considered smarter and their ways were awarded and highly respected.

There have been, and are, exceptions, of course, where a school's curriculum has been attentive to diverse learners. But the institutional values of the public and educational systems in general favor the students with a Linear brainstyle.

The ways of others who learned and achieved their goals in any way other than the traditional Linear way were frequently considered to be doing things in the "wrong" way and/or have been labeled disordered.

It was also a time in history when a kinesthetic apprenticeship education carried less status than a Linear-based, academic education. Gone were the days of apprenticeships for professional careers. Experience no longer counted as a door opener for those with high skill levels but no formal degree credentials.

More and more top-notch professionals—educators, counselors, librarians, engineers, and many more with decades of experience—were forced to work under newly graduated, licensed individuals who knew less about the job. Hands-on internships were tacked onto academic training to provide a smattering of direct experience. But the problem was that some people couldn't get through the academic material and testing in order to prove themselves in their field of interest.

I'll never forget meeting Doug, who was rated by his peers to be the best tugboat crew member on Long Island Sound. He subbed for the captain when needed and wanted to become credentialed as a licensed captain now that he'd turned eighteen and had the prerequisite years of experience running the boats. This meant he had to pass a multiple-choice paper-and-pencil test.

As with many people who have ADD characteristics, he could demonstrate the skills required of the job, but passing a paper-and-pencil test about what he knew was nearly impossible. Doug had one more chance to pass the test.

His story did end well, for he passed it on the fifth and last try. But does it make sense to be judged in such a way?

It was at this time, 1996, that I first began to sense an analogy forming in my mind between race, gender, and styles of learning. College and university Linear-style education had increasingly been on the rise to prominence over trade-school education. It had been a time when diversity issues were wending their way through our society's consciousness.

By then I could see the ADD brainstyle taking a similar value-laden path that race and gender had followed. The word diversity increasingly haunted my thinking about ADD. Brainstyle as an issue of diversity gnawed at me.

My perspective on the style of processing information fell in line with a similar diversity model that was free of judgments as applied to individuals and institutional parameters.

I realized that the breadth of jobs, professions, and the ways of life in which you can find a place for yourself ranges broadly depending in part upon the type of ADD and the balance of ADD and Linear traits that your brain has available to use, along with finding the right *fit* for yourself.

But at this time, I wasn't yet emotionally confident and strong enough to fully stand up for what I believed. That has changed. I now have more experience and personal power to stand by the beliefs that simply won't go away.

I needed time to assess many more people and situations to check my own perspective of ADD as it affected the people with whom I worked. I needed to understand the differences of what I was thinking, as I compared my view with the view of the majority of professionals of the time.

The long time it took to own what I initially came to know intuitively served a purpose. I needed that time to go beyond a "right" and "wrong," "me" and "them" mentality. Instead, different beliefs needed to be acknowledged. I realized there is room for a wide variance in beliefs not just in religion, but also in medicine, politics, and education. There are, after all, as many ways to believe as there are people who declare their beliefs and accept another's beliefs. I didn't know it then, but by the mid-1990s, I had begun to think seriously about ADD as a diversity issue.

INTRODUCING ADD AS A DIVERSITY ISSUE

When I look back on the next set of formative years, 1997 to 2005, it is now clear to me that I played out a sequence of professional activities that reinforced the idea of ADD as a diversity issue. Prior to that time, I was leaving the idea of ADD as a medical condition and "coming to" the idea of ADD as a nonpathological sociocultural difference in the brainstyles of people with the attributes called ADD, shown in table 1.1.

My writing, training, and speaking helped me to further extend the perspectives I'd come to earlier. I began to notice how the different ones of us *fit* or didn't *fit* in the work we did. On the one hand, our ADD caused all kinds of stress and trouble. On the other, our ADD made us good at what we did.

When the *fit* was poor, adjustments in the workplace, such as diverse organizational skill-building in an ADD way, made all the difference. Gone were the long-term projects that had to be accomplished one step at a time toward the development of a five-year plan. In its place those involved worked with the understanding that they could use their big-picture organizational skills to accomplish a desired outcome. Brainstorming and weaving together of errant bits and pieces of analogous information and resources became the fodder for feeding the development of patterns and

Table 1.1. ADD Attributes

Attribute	Description
The Big Picture	Many of us see the big picture before we see or make use of any of the details that make it up. Usually creative by nature, "big picture" people often see a complete vision of what we want to achieve before we start moving toward our goals. In fact, we don't travel well to any goal unless we are provided with the big picture to begin with. We often also put together groups of patterns and relationships and build upon how the goal is going to function as seen in the final vision.
Patterns and Relationships (Way of Viewing)	We pay attention to the patterns and relationships within the big picture. Our focus of attention tends to be on the relationship between details rather than on the details themselves. We first see the interconnections and patterns that are formed between things and groups of similarly functioning groups of details, rather than the elements that make them up.
Function (How Things Function)	If we are to know how to proceed toward a goal, we must know its purpose. How is this goal to be used? Rather than seeing the details that make up the task, we see the function the details play. Then we can know the steps to take to achieve the goal.
Kinesthetic Learner	We naturally learn through the process of doing something, rather than by reading or listening about whatever we are learning. We write a book to learn to write. We don't learn to write a book by studying about writing a book, doing exercises or worksheets, or taking exams so we can then write a book. We are totally and completely able to learn any subject or body of professional material, no matter how complex, by utilizing (hands on) kinesthetic learning. That's why the apprenticeship model works well for us.
High Level of Activity (Mentally, Physically, Emotionally, and Verbally)	Naturally invested with lots of energy, we learn, create, and produce best when we are active. Our innate skills seek environments for expression that allow us to be physically active and verbally expressive. Our minds are curious and exploring and often work at lightning speed. After all, remember, we see the big picture first—so we don't need to slowly progress from one detail to another in order to reach that completed picture. We're also aided by our rapid awareness of the patterns that often give us early clues about the journey we are taking. The icing on the cake is the presence of big, broad, expressive emotions that communicate to us and others with clarity.
Sensitive (In Relation to All the Senses)	Our sensitivity is felt through our senses: sight, sound, taste, smell, and touch as well as intuition. Extremely empathetic, our sensors are calibrated finely. Liken us to the dog that hears sound not perceived by the human ear. We sense a level that not all people have available to them. We are empathic

(continued)

Table 1.1. *Continued*

Attribute	Description
	and responsive to our environments. We can be wounded when others do not see or sense the source of the wounding, yet we experience it nonetheless. When a companion has a feeling such as anger, we know it even if the person is unaware of it and denies it. Many of us are psychic, though we may not be comfortable with this skill or may not purposely use it.
Responsiveness	Because we are so sensitive and tend to act kinesthetically when attempting to reach a goal, we tend to be seen as reactive. With a wide range of emotions, readily experiencing joy and pain, we often express our feelings and do something about situations that others do not even know exist.
Sensate (An Inner Knowing)	We tend to think first through our ability to sense what is going on rather than by thinking about something that is happening or needed. We simply *know*, having an inner sensory vision, experience, or intuition. We often feel the sensing physically in our bodies. Once we've perceived an event on a sensory level, we can decide what to do in response. We even store information using this mechanism rather than by categorizing according to the labels in more general use.
Rhythmic Timing/Nature (A Natural Sensing)	Rather than responding to an arbitrary scheme to keep track of time, we tend to use natural rhythms and our own internal timing to get things done. We can apply this skill to a project or to getting the rest our bodies need. We may work at night and sleep in the daytime. We may naturally eat at times that vary from a three-meal-a-day schedule. We rarely break projects down into equal time segments in order to get them done by a certain time—but rather work when we feel creative and don't work when we feel unwilling or hesitant. When our innate timing is allowed to blossom and we are trained to recognize it, we nearly always get things done on time.
Inner Locus of Perception and Control (Related to Sensing)	Our worldview comes from within ourselves. Our ability to organize, work with time and timing, maintain control over our behavior, and do whatever we need to do is idiosyncratically guided from within ourselves rather than from the outside culture, community, or other people, including their laws and socially accepted customs. We will choose to follow the laws even when we disagree with them, but consciously seek alternatives to change the laws to match up with our inner beliefs. We know and sense and can learn to live in a responsible way that yields the same results achieved by our more Linear counterparts if we follow what feels right to us. We know what to do by listening to our inner drumbeat, not by using a template produced outside of ourselves into which we are expected to *fit*.

functions for their projects. With a hands-on approach, the ADD players created an outcome that pleased those working together.

The goals of Analogue and Linear individuals and teams could be the same. It was only that the processes of reaching the goals were different, depending upon the diverse brain construction of those involved.

Early on it became apparent to me that a person didn't *have* ADD, but had more or fewer ADD *attributes*. I saw a continuum in my mind that ran from all Linear attributes on one end to all Analogue attributes on the other. (See figure 1.1.)

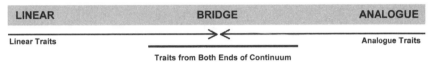

LINEAR	BRIDGE	ANALOGUE
Linear Traits	Traits from Both Ends of Continuum	Analogue Traits

Figure 1.1.

On the far end of the Analogue side of the scale, a person will primarily have ADD brainstyle attributes. But as people have fewer ADD traits and more Linear traits they will move toward the Linear side of the scale. Moving through the middle of the scale will yield Bridge people who are fairly balanced in the two brainstyle types. There's a similar pattern for people with a primarily Linear style of brain construction. Thus, no one "has ADD," but has more or fewer ADD traits or more or fewer Linear traits.

With this in mind, I saw how people could help one another personally, as well as in the workplace, by mixing and matching their diverse brainstyles, be they ADD or Linear or a mixture of both.

Linear folks can help Analogue people either by assisting them to accommodate to the world of the Linear or by filling in the gaps to the Linear world for them—a team approach in action. And in reverse, the Analogue people can equally play a valuable role with their Linear counterparts.

Having someone on your team to provide the support you need until you become stronger and more confident is a great gift. New doorways to discover what you like and don't like will kindle the growth of your ultimate goal: creating an environment for your

True Self that *fits* you. Mixing and matching of interests and skills provides you with as many opportunities to learn about yourself by disliking what you're being exposed to as liking it. Even neutrality serves a purpose as you watch your reactions to the things to which you're exposed.

As the role of ADD worked its way into the world of diversity and vice versa, I found myself becoming increasingly interested in the phenomenal contributions the outcome was contributing to relationships, workplace settings, social institutions, and the culture at large.

More and more I became convinced that it was not necessary to "get rid of" the effects of ADD. I realized we can choose to find ways to accommodate how we fit our brainstyle. We each must find our own special combination of talents and individualized gifts that make us up. The result is that we utilize the talents and subsequent opportunities we desire and leave a footprint more than twice the size and value we could leave with only one footprint that we think is flawed.

CONFIRMING MY PERSPECTIVE

Let me share three success stories of the kind that confirmed my perspective. Each person's success story contained magic—the magic of feelings. Exposing feelings while following their dreams gave them the opportunity to learn and grow from others who traveled by their side. By seeing in another person what they were feeling, they were better able to face their fears and doubts in order to express their ADD selves.

Milele's Magic

In the beginning, Milele's story didn't sound very magical or a good candidate for success. She was the oldest of eight children with an alcoholic father who abused her mother, a mother who died when Milele was nearing the end of her first term as a college senior. She said, "I was a senior in college on Friday afternoon and head of a household with five kids to raise on Sunday. My stepfather left right after my mama's funeral and wasn't heard of until he died ten years later."

Not a terribly hopeful beginning for a woman whose journey to her magic lay in her future. What got her through these hard times? She chuckled and said, "I was too ornery to quit. I'd always had a mission to 'save' people, even in elementary school, and once I discovered the ravages of unrecognized ADD, I knew how to make it beyond my impulsivity, problems with attention, and restlessness. Once I discovered our family's ADD heritage, I made it my business to learn all I could about what to do.

"My success is shaped by the way in which my brain is made: my ability to read people, and work with them, my wonderful intuitive ability to sense others—their feelings, capabilities, hopes, and dreams. I also instinctively know what they have to overcome in order to reach their potential. All the good talents I have are because of my ADD brain. Above all, I've learned to learn from my mistakes so I don't repeat the mishaps of an earlier time."

Finally, Milele wants others to know: "The reality is that I've always had this ADD, I always will have ADD, and there is freedom to live with ADD." She continues with a recommendation to all: "Consume all the experience and knowledge you can. Use it when you're able!"

Thus Speaketh a Healed Healer! Cesario's Magic

In the beginning, Cesario described himself as "a young person who has to go out to learn." Smiling softly, he continued, "Take, for example, where a young person goes out and has a beer or something like that. That's going without thinking. Anyone can go without thinking. Maybe they try to do it again. Maybe all the thinking they are doing is thinking about what they are going to do."

At the time, he was in the Navy. "I wasn't doing anything good. The things I was supposed to be doing, I wasn't getting done. So I quit drinking cold turkey. I stopped. That wasn't for me," he said.

Something in his Native American soul knew truth that bode well for him to follow the tradition of his people. I wondered how and why he and his wife ended up back at the pueblo after they were married. His answer came in story form, as did most of his answers to questions.

"I was standing there on the deck of the ship and the question occurred to me: 'What am I doing here fighting somebody's war, and my people are in the United States fighting the United States government, trying to fight to get back our land?' That's kind of what brought me back here—to do what I could do."

Cesario's magic of feelings was imbedded in the culture in which he was raised on the reservation. His story—and the story of his people—is not dissimilar to the story of ADD people who have been stripped of their power to learn, work, and express themselves freely using their innate ADD way. Although the term ADD was not used in talking with Cesario, his ADD way of thinking *fit* the life that he carved out for himself and his family.

He also managed to overcome the effects of some of the potential handicaps of ADD by choosing a companion who had the skills to organize paperwork and keep up with it, and who has been willing to work with him. His choices came to him naturally because he trusted the *True Self* within him. He recognized how he was made and placed his attention in that direction, saying, "I gotta be out there doing something, something that I can see that it's kind of growing, or train a horse, or teach a person or help somebody. That's me."

And that's the acceptance by each person in the culture of his ancestors, a culture sadly fragmented in today's world, but one being resuscitated by members of the current generation like Cesario.

More power to these teachers, leaders, and role models as they say, "We must all walk our talk."

Jeannine's and Kevin's Magic

Jeannine is a gentle soul who was introduced to drugs as a child in order to pay attention for long periods of time so she could do the load of ironing assigned to her by a very sensitive mother, a dreamer caught in the trap of being a teenaged mother with no way to "get out" to reach her own dreams. She didn't mean harm. She just didn't know how to deal with her angry, violent husband. She didn't know how to accomplish the dream of having a big beautiful house and get an education.

The result is that Jeannine didn't have a "happy childhood." In addition, she was called "stupid." It seems she had learning disabilities that went unnoticed in the 1950s, as well as behavior problems resulting from her dysfunctional home life.

In contrast, Kevin's early years were spent as an only child on a farm with grandparents. He loved it. "I was irrigating the field when I was seven. I drove tractors and generally was free to do everything, even though it drove my grandfather crazy." But then, his grandpa taught him to drive and laughed a lot.

Kevin grew up knowing that he and his family were "all ADD." Extremely hyperactive, he was comfortable being how he was, loving to play and joke around, and go, go, go. Comfortable, that is, until he had to go to school regularly and he was with his mother more of the time. His mom was not eager to embrace the whole idea of ADD, Kevin said. She told him, "You're crazy, Kevin. There ain't none of us sick but you."

Kevin tried to defend himself. "I tried to explain to her. 'It's like, Mom, you don't understand. This ain't something I grew into.'" At that, he demonstrated how he reached out with his hand, grabbing a bunch of air. Then he continued, "I told her, 'This came in my genes. Your genes.'"

After this exchange he was secluded and left out of the family. He was put off in a corner or left alone because he couldn't sit still. In school he could do math in his way, but not the way the teacher was making her students do it. He couldn't keep his attention on the blackboard. "I would know the answers as soon as the teacher wrote the problems on the board. But she called me 'defiant,' after which I was labeled 'Oppositional Defiant.'"

Kevin, like Jeannine, was what I call "undereducated," which means much smarter than they have the education to reflect.

Both Kevin and Jeannine began to turn their lives around when they met a "special other person" with whom they made a relationship. For Jeannine, a friend recommended she go to an ashram in Arizona. It took her a month to actually move into it, but it was there that she met her husband "and began to shed who I was," she said.

Over the years, she worked on her learning problems and the emotional residue left by her early life experiences. Sweetly, she confides, "My husband tells me every day, 'If you died today, you did it, you made it, you hit the summit, you made the top of the mountain because you broke the cycle of your childhood.'"

Miles away, Kevin met Deb. Deb knew how to make a living and balance her finances. In fact, she was so competent that she never sought help and didn't receive it as a matter of course. So Deb was emotionally lonely, having been on her own since she was a teen.

Meeting a man like Kevin, who was younger than she but full of life and playfulness, touched a part of Deb that had never felt warm. She was hungry to be loved. And Kevin loved making her smile. Slowly, Deb got used to his sweet attention and loving behavior and felt whole for the first time in her life.

As Kevin realized how much Deb valued him, he felt like he'd been given the moon. And he felt valuable for the first time in his life. But in contrast, Deb felt that Kevin had given life. She began to realize her true value.

Deb's and Jeannine's husbands continually gave their partners the magic needed for each of them to begin the journey to believe in themselves and eventually to find their *True Selves*. Milele's involvement with self-help and educational environments did much the same for her as she learned and learned and learned from everyone and everything around her. After all, do we who teach often not learn more from what we are passing on to our students than our students learn from us?

As I said before sharing the stories of Milele, Cesario, and Kevin and Jeannine, there's no more necessity to think about getting rid of the effects of ADD. They each accommodated the way in which they could find a fit for their brainstyle. We each must find our special combination of talents and individualized gifts that make us up. The result is that we utilize our talents and subsequent opportunities to advantage.

To find your way to your magic—the magic of feelings—you must expose your feelings, at least to yourself. One way to do that is to follow your dreams by investigating new opportunities. Perhaps you can get an idea from Cesario, who brought the strong energy of his culture into play even as he was living away from the reservation that subsequently drew him home. He listened to his feelings and knew when he was making a right choice.

Seek and find models who will inspire you. In today's world, you may do information interviewing with individuals who are living or working within a setting that is new to you. Or you may benefit from volunteer internships that will guide you to a fitting future.

In a way, this is what Jeannine did when she checked out a retreat setting in Arizona and discovered a way of life that she hadn't known about. There, with the support of the man who became her husband—a man who believed more in her than she ever dreamed was possible—Jeannine started to recognize who she might become. Twenty-six years later, she had not only reached her *True Self* but had gone way beyond anything that she could have imagined.

You never know who is traveling a path nearby you from whom you can gain support or be exposed to what resonates for you. By seeing in another person what you are feeling, you are better able to face your fears and doubts as you gently begin to express your ADD self.

Of course, be cautious about being wooed by illusions and fantasies created in relation to certain job situations or environments. It's rather like going on a vacation where you are served or relax in the sunshine with little to do to get your own needs met; there are no toilets to scrub and no grocery shopping to do while the kids are clamoring for chips during rush-hour traffic.

An attentive host or welcoming hostess is not the same as someone with whom you spend hour upon hour upon day working side by side. The future fantasies created at that time are questionable at least and may have little grounding in the long run. Watch out if you are quite creative of mind. You'll need to ground yourself to the realities of daily living before casting the lot of your *True Self* into the situation. Note it. Enjoy it. Consider it. And let time go by living it day to day to see what the lasting power of the environment feels like to you in the long run.

One last word of warning! Please be cautious about being wooed by the illusions created when someone is trying to convince you how wonderful a particular job offer is. If you choose a path you think will make you more valuable, or if you think the job will pay more or make you popular, but it doesn't make you *happy*, you're likely to shortchange yourself. Do what is in the heart of your *True Self*, the true indicator of what is right for you.

In this way, you will not only likely *be* a success, you'll *feel* like a success.

THE MAGIC OF DIVERSITY: THE RELATIONSHIP BETWEEN ANALOGUE AND LINEAR BRAINSTYLES

Finally in the key years of 1997 to 2005, I began to realize the incredible need to utilize the full range of potential brain construction. That means a full range of ADD attributes as well as Linear ones: People working together, teaming, and partnering to bring their unique attributes to bear for the greater cause, individual, family, and community. All forms, styles, and interests are needed if the end product, service, or outcome of your work is to reach its apex. Only years later, do I understand the importance of the relationship between ADD attributes and non-ADD attributes as a means to creating true success in our culture.

The opportunity to consult in the minimum security federal correctional institution in Bastrop, Texas—identifying and helping ADD inmates, and later providing ADD education and training for the prison staff—led me to the hands-on field experience I thrived upon to raise my insight into the relationship between the Linear and Analogue brainstyles.

Through my work in the prison, I met Dr. John Rubel, PsyD, a board-certified psychologist who is about as Linear as they come. We immediately clicked when he served cappuccinos from the machine in his office. What a rare exception to my previous history with seriously Linear clinicians! We each reached as far as we could toward the other's brainstyle language system, perceptual understanding, and ways of teaching, counseling, and preparing, as well as presenting, material for classes of inmates.

We grew into a high level of trust with one another, even though neither of us was able to fully connect with the explanations, expressions, and presentations of the other's brainstyles. We seemed to sense which one of us would start the orientation of a topic. And we would also know when to turn the presentation over to the other. We were guided by knowing whether the topic lent itself to a Linear presentation or an Analogue one. As a result, inmate groups, made up of both ADD and Linear men, were able to see firsthand how to reach across brainstyle differences to work with someone different from themselves. From the beginning I didn't observe or think of ADD as something I or you might "have" or not "have," but that we might have more or fewer attributes. As I continued my work, I began to pay more attention to the Linear attributes that my colleagues, friends, and those with whom I worked clinically bore.

I'll never forget one presentation at the University of Michigan in the mid-1990s. I was opening an ADD conference by highlighting some fairly standard attributes of ADD, such as "getting off track" and "ignoring the details of a job." I found myself making jokes about how those with a Linear brainstyle, unlike us ADD folks, had problems too. I said they had Goal Surplus Disorder (GSD), when too much time was spent on reaching a goal to the exclusion of perceiving and understanding the process leading to the goal, and Color Commentary Deficiency (CCD) when they presented facts about a situation without using any background words of interest to describe the event. The audience laughed loudly, with both ADD and non-ADD people taking the comments in stride.

The experience probably only lasted a couple of minutes. But, it made an impression on me—one I've never forgotten. I saw how people with the whole range of brainstyles could work together and laugh together without having to claim that "the others" had something "wrong" with them. I had an inkling of how we might become a team with mutual respect for one another.

"GIRLS' WEEKEND OUT" (LATER RENAMED "BRAIN DIVERSITY WORKSHOP")

About the same time that I was wanting to understand more about the similarities and differences between brainstyles, several friends in my local community also wanted to know about their brainstyle makeup. So "Girls' Weekend Out" was created.

With coffee and snacks in hand, we sat on the patio of a lake cottage in central Texas, and I immediately began to realize three natural breakdowns in the group of Texas women with me. The continuum I'd sensed began to show itself. I gave everyone an ADD checklist, and that yielded scores from "few" to "some" to "many" ADD attributes. (You can find that checklist at the end of this chapter, if you're interested in trying it out for yourself.)

Ranging in age from thirty-seven to fifty-six, the participants were interested in all sorts of self-recognition measures and parameters that would help them see themselves from varying angles. We utilized personality measures, learning and brainstyle checklists, social-emotional scores, and listings of educational achievements. And we talked and talked, sharing likes and dislikes. Each one of us shared a short family history and life-dreams wish list.

Once we finished this sharing period, we divided into fairly equal groups of Linear, Bridge, and Analogue individuals. The Linear and Analogue individuals anchored the ends of the continuum with an equal number of people in the middle serving as "bilingual" Bridge people.

Bridge people were those who had both ADD and Linear attributes. This was the first time I had really spent time thinking about the Bridge group as I saw it manifest in front of my eyes that weekend. The power and skill set of this group continues to amaze me as they are the ones who can translate between us ADD "Big Picture" go-to-Chicago-from-Dallas-via-Florida people and the Linear one-step-at-a- time, check-every-minute-detail-of-a-plan-before-expressing-a-preference-much-less-acting-upon-it people. Oh my, do we ever need them as translators and mediators in our world of brainstyle differences.

The women expressed little confusion or concern about who identified with which of the three labels. By dividing participants into three groups using their scores, it seemed that a natural breakdown evolved. In retrospect, I wonder more today at how that relates to the reporting of percentages of ADD people in our society. If ADD is seen more as a style than a discreet "condition," perhaps it's not so strange. As you've no doubt figured out, I am more likely to believe the introspective perceptions of the people who are being studied in this regard than an observer with a different brainstyle trying to label someone.

At our "Girls' Weekend Out" we began the first of a number of assignments that led us to understand ourselves and our different brainstyles, one that you can replicate in your own arena of influence.

In Round 1, each of the three groups was assigned the same task. First, I purposely chose a task that clearly required Linear attributes to achieve because it would be the simplest to describe and implement. The tasks were not time limited. No one felt rushed. When two of the three groups had reached completion, only a limited amount of additional time was allowed before we stopped the round to view the results.

The assignment required the members of the group to order themselves by the size of their shoes.

It took the seven Linear women about one minute to sort themselves into a clearly observable outcome. They stood up, formed a line with the woman having the longest shoe size standing on the left and then, one by one, they simply called out their shoe size and took their place in line with the smallest shoe size falling at the right end of the line.

The Bridge group used about three or four minutes to complete the assigned task. They talked more about what they were doing, sat down to swing their feet forward comparing shoes, and made comments about the shoes they were wearing. Someone said, "I always had the biggest feet of anyone I knew." Someone else added, "Well, we'll just have to see about that." They all laughed and quickly shared their sizes and were ready to report the results. They didn't, however line up, either by standing or switching chairs, to demonstrate their foot size in a seriated manner.

The third group broke out of the circle in which the group had been sitting and moved to cushioned chairs outside the ring. A couple of women sat on the arms of a couch, while one woman sat on the floor. They all began to talk, and a low buzz of words could be heard all around the room. They weren't rude or thoughtless, but every now and again a laugh would emerge to a level that the others in the room looked over to see what was happening. Invariably, smiles came to the faces of those noticing the ADD group's obvious fun-making.

Moving over so I could hear the conversation that was going on, I overheard comments about first prom shoes, most embarrassing time in high heels, and the trials and tribulations of toe abnormalities. Do I need to tell you that we shut down the exercise without group three ever having reached the goal of the assignment?

The ADD participants reported in their summary of the workshop that they totally understood the point of the exercise and got more out of it than if they'd stood in line like the Linear people did. They recognized as much or more about the differences between Linear and ADD styles of brain construction than any of the others in the workshop. Interestingly, they seemed to understand more about the big picture style of ADD brain construction in contrast to a Linear construction and much preferred their way.

They generally liked the way they were made, only wanting help with specific situations that caused them trouble when a Linear brainstyle was required or demanded in order to demonstrate that they had achieved a goal—even when they could demonstrate goal achievement by demonstrating it. They wanted to be able to show what they could do, not be tested about it.

These workshops had an enormous impact on me as I became more and more certain that depathologizing ADD was important. I was beginning to learn how much we individuals with differences need one another. We make up a whole—a whole that brings a full round of perceptions that can lead to a complete picture of whatever is being viewed and a more balanced outcome and solution to problems or creations with which we are being confronted.

One more insight must be given space at this time, fitting in as it does to the continuum-building section of this history. It happened during another "Girls' Weekend Out" workshop. What made this one different was the feedback from one of the participants at the end of the day, adding to my understanding of the continuum aspect of ADD as a diversity issue.

Melissa, a sales and marketing professional, was able to clearly express what she had experienced as a member of the Bridge group during the assignment that required her group to design a public presentation piece about ADD. The assignment had been for each of the three groups to find a means by which they could draw the public to an event that would demonstrate brainstyle differences.

The Linear group had come up with a perfectly worded flyer announcing an informational public meeting about brainstyle differences. Finished and ready to go in under twenty minutes, they even made plans for where to hang the flyers.

The ADD group had designed a skit in which they would act out the differences between Linear and Analogue styles through a comedy routine presented at the local theater. They had not, however, written down the dialogue, nor did they have plans to practice the skit further. They did not consider how to check whether the theater was available at the same time they wanted to schedule the production, nor consider advertising to attract an audience. Rather than planning about costumes and props, they simply said to one another, "Wear what you want."

Everyone loved the skit, applauded, and thought it was a great idea—an idea, though, that might not get any further without help from others with a different brainstyle.

The last group to report was the Bridge group. Initially they were excited about this assignment. They weren't, however, able to fully complete the task in the twenty-minute allotted time. Melissa helped us understand why, despite initial interest, they didn't fully produce what was expected.

She reported how at first she and many of her Bridge cohorts had thought about a flyer but then felt it wouldn't be compelling enough to draw a receptive audience, especially an audience made up of people with an Analogue style of brain construction. More than that, she strongly felt the tug of the artistic side within her that wanted, yearned, to do something more creative than to give a straightforward verbal program announcement.

No sooner had this feeling flooded through her than she and the others were tugged back toward feeling they should just get something ready in the time provided. But then again, the pull returned from her creative side wanting to accomplish something cool. All that tugging and pulling ate up time so that they didn't finish in twenty minutes. When we told them it was okay to take an extra few minutes, they created a truly lovely, effective invitation for the public called "Girls' Night Out Workshop" and subtitled, "Why We Think and Act the Way We Do" with delightful graphics that they had the skills to create. They even planned who would do the art and when it would be accomplished prior to the distribution of the pamphlets and flyers.

Melissa spoke about feeling guilty at times because she had wanted to help make something really good, because of her background in sales and marketing. She wanted to use her creative talents to express how good she had been feeling because of attending the workshop. But, when there didn't seem to be time to be creative, she thought she and the others in her group should get a simple, quick announcement ready. Yet she and others in the group couldn't let go of the desire to create something that would reach out and pull people in. This tug and push—being affected by the beliefs associated with the Linear side of her mind and the desires associated with the ADD part of her mind—set her up for frustration. Then, when the Bridge group was given the extra time, a thing of beauty emerged—well worth the time.

ADD 101 FOR PRISON ADMINISTRATORS, TEACHERS, AND GUARDS

A final experience that helped me formulate my ideas of ADD was also provided by the federal correctional institution at Bastrop,

Texas. A workshop was designed to supply information and training for approximately thirty-five guards, administrators, teachers,
and clinicians, called "ADD 101 for Prison Administrators, Teachers, and Guards." It was based upon the original "Brain Diversity
Workshop" and highlighted two different lessons about ADD—
lessons that had not been apparent to me before the training.

Dr. Rubel and I became aware that we needed to provide
information and skill-building to staff responsible for working
with inmates who probably had ADD attributes—attributes that
added to their difficulty in adjusting to prison life. Using the
ADD checklist, we discovered that more than half of the staff
participants had either a large or moderately high number of
Linear traits. Fewer than ten had a high number of ADD attributes. Those who did tended to be guards who taught classes
with the prisoners such as GED, shop classes in which prisoners
build furniture and toys for children, and horticulture and gar-
dening that used the prison grounds as their field setting. These
teachers tended to have a higher number of ADD attributes than
the administrative participants.

The first unexpected discovery made during the workshop surprised me. Whenever Analogue tasks were given to participants
who had few Analogue traits, they developed responses (symptoms) that were identical to the ADD symptoms listed in the *Diagnostic and Statistical Manual of Mental Disorders (DSM)* of the
American Psychiatric Association. They demonstrated symptoms
of ADD. These included poor impulse control, temper and impatience, hypersensitivity, argumentativeness, and blaming behavior.
The Linear participants failed to finish the Analogue tasks, demonstrated a poor attention span, became hyperactive or restless,
were easily distracted, clowned around, and became judgmental
and critical as their stress grew. The tasks didn't *fit* their brainstyle.

When the Linear group was assigned a closing Analogue task to
present to the whole group, they failed miserably. The assignment
was to spontaneously design a show-and-tell community presentation that would demonstrate the ADD-way of effective commu-

nication. What they wrote on the chalkboard made little sense to any of the ADD or Bridge participants. It neither hung together as a teaching unit nor did it capture an effective teaching mode or style for the audience to learn from.

While they would have been candidates for a grade of "F" in a regular classroom, the more serious difficulty was that the Linear people in the room had no idea how inadequate their product was. They only saw target words that they knew and they thought the use of the words meant the teaching process had been accomplished. As a community teaching tool, there was little to no evidence that communication of the function of the program design was achieved.

MORE DISCOVERIES

The second discovery that Linear participants had difficulty understanding was how Nonlinear individuals in our group used their talents and abilities to learn and process information, problem solve, and reach goals using their innate ADD style. They simply couldn't make sense of it, tending to discount the validity of the Nonlinear responses and outcomes. The ADD way was simply considered *wrong*.

This includes: learning kinesthetically; using intuition and inner senses to plan, organize, and make sense of what is happening around us; and seeing the big picture as a starting point for planning, while leaving the details for later inclusion—*after* they had formed the details into patterns or saw the function of the groupings on the way to the goal. The Linear participants could not imagine not having a detailed outline before starting the construction or development of a project nor developing an outline for what had already been done. They tried to understand functioning with multiple track awareness rather than doing one thing at a time; working more effectively by walking around, changing activities frequently, and having a radio or some activity in the background in order to be able to work continuously on a project. But they just could not.

Playing around and using humor in the early stages of creative work, such as designing a program to communicate to new staff about ADD, acts as a benefit. More originality tends to occur for ADD people and a high level of attention gets the job done in a timely manner. These behaviors and processes were over-whelmingly difficult for people with a primary Linear thinking brainstyle to understand.

To help those of us who are not very Linear oriented, I'll share an example that comes to mind to demonstrate that ADD folks are not the only brainstyle that has difficulty doing tasks that don't *fit* them. At the time that I was writing *ADD and Creativity* in the mid-1990s, I started an ADD and Creativity group at my of-fice. People interested in, or working in, the arts were joined by educators and university students who wanted to broaden their understanding of brainstyles and the arts.

I recall having a university student come to my office who clearly demonstrated the issue of *fit*. She was an education major who carried a 4.0 GPA in her senior year. Nearing graduation, she was required to attend a creative writing class at school. Her professor sent her to my group as a part of the classwork.

Upon arriving, each participant filled out an ADD checklist to give a rough idea of where they lay on the brainstyle continuum. The student, prim and precise, filled out the form and immedi-ately began to complain about the waste of time of having to take the creative writing class. She thought it foolish to play around with words and not write in prescribed ways. She found specific poetic forms such as writing sonnets acceptable, but not writing in free-form.

When we got to the part of the group where participants were to write a short creative assignment to be followed by a period of sharing how it felt and what difficulties or pleasures each par-ticipant experienced in relationship to her brainstyle, the student walked out of the group, proclaiming that it was a real waste of time for any serious student.

That student scored on the high Linear end of the continuum when the checklist was scored. She apparently had a difficult time understanding how to make an "A" in her mandated creative writing class and feared losing her 4.0 GPA. I often wondered about her later and hoped that she would find a setting that could appreciate her skills and be gentle with her when she was required to enter the world of the Analogue processor.

Here's what we can learn from the former examples about anyone who is required to function in an arena calling for skills that are opposite of their brainstyle. It is difficult, if not impossible to function up to par when our brainstyle doesn't *fit* an assigned task. We become anxious, feel guilty, and want to escape as a result. Our emotional system reacts negatively to the requirements and we suffer fear and/or wounding as a result.

I know from myriad ADD people I've met with that they suffer greatly when required to work in a Linear way, and in contrast often achieve quality results when allowed to accomplish the same tasks in an Analogue way that *fits* them.

I'm interested in the reactions of people who score high on the Linear scale demonstrating the same "symptoms" as ADD people score when being required to do a task that is an Analogue task. In contrast, the women's group participants did not become symptomatic in the few situations I observed. They tended to be intrigued by the differences rather than distressed by the differences. They did not tend to judge their own or other's goal achievement levels. But then, this was a voluntary group—free of competition, grades, or specific requirements.

Also variable are an individual's responses. Dr. Rubel, prison psychologist, was and continues to be comfortable around Analogue tasks. In fact he says he purposely seeks them out to broaden his life experiences. His life is primarily structured in a Linear way. His play still looks fairly Linear to me, but he tends to reach toward new types of interests and to people who are significantly different from him in brainstyle. As we work together, Linear is his turf and Analogue is mine. We simply seek to find a middle-ground language that allows us to be mutually understood, or as mentioned earlier, we simply concede to the other one as necessary to achieve a result that we cannot achieve together.

The Linear college student, however, did not have the power to avoid the Analogue task and so became stressed as many ADD learners do in attempting to complete Linear tasks. As the stress rises, so do the "symptom" responses that are considered pathological by the *DSM*.

From these experiences, I came to see how there is a continuum of natural brainstyles from those that are predominantly Linear to those that are predominantly Analogue in nature. As we visualize the continuum from one extreme to the other, we progress through a middle section that is mixed, which I've called the Bridge people brainstyle, where we find those who have a mixture of the two extremes. Each has its strengths.

Traits associated with every part of the spectrum studied have value—from Analogue through Linear. But no one part of the continuum can do all things. Together, however, people can bring their strengths and skills to bear, joining with one another so that the end result is balanced and complete with the best of both worlds contributing what each has to offer.

There is simply no room in this model for devaluing one aspect of the human continuum of brainstyles. Perhaps it is time to put aside shortsighted, judgmental criticism and the pathologizing of brainstyles and, instead, celebrate the diversity of what the whole of our population brings to make the world a better place. Devaluation of one aspect of human differences reflects self-centered, prejudicial thinking. It truly does take all kinds of people to make up a thriving, creative, progressive society in which all are seen as valuable and all are provided for—no winners and losers. With this kind of thinking, everyone wins!

There is no doubt in my mind: Attention Deficit Disorder is a diversity issue.

ADD Assessment Checklist

I am including this list here because I think you might be interested in it. People sometimes enjoy seeing whether or not they recognize themselves in this checklist. People with an ADD style of brain construction often identify with many of these traits. The higher your score, the more likely you are to be ADD.

Answer the following questions about yourself. If you've spent time learning to accommodate the situation or feeling, reference your answer to a time before you did your self-work. You may also find it helpful to have someone else answer these questions in relation to you.

	Yes	Some	No
Do you often fail to finish detailed tasks?			
Do you have trouble managing your checkbook and finances?			
Are you easily distracted when dealing with details, paper work, and administrative tasks?			
Do you get bored doing repetitive tasks?			
Do you get bored or lose attention with sustained-action tasks?			
Do you rarely do careful long-term planning, even with major decisions?			
Have you teamed up with people who manage details and organize for you?			
Do you feel you've achieved below your potential in school or at work?			
Do you frequently act without thinking?			
Do you multi-task, doing more than one thing at a time?			
Do you work better when shifting from one activity to another?			
Do you have many interests that you enjoy for a while, then drop, regardless of financial investment?			
Have you struggled with substance abuse?			
Do you respond better to being asked than told?			
Do you have a sense of humor?			
Do your eyes twinkle?			
Do you call and talk out, interrupting conversations?			
Do you get restless waiting your turn in a group situation?			

(continued)

ADD Assessment Checklist

	Yes	Some	No
Do you feel impatient or express your impatience with boring or slow-moving situations?			
Is it hard for you to structure your environment or projects?			
Does your creativity feel cramped by too much structure?			
Do you often finish another's sentence?			
Do you prefer activity over stillness most of the time?			
Do you become sleepy or restless if not active?			
Is it hard for you to sit still?			
Is it hard for you to stay seated?			
Have you frequently changed jobs regardless of the reason?			
Do you think better when you're active?			
Have you often had periods of depression?			
Are you very sensitive emotionally?			
Do you take things personally or get your feelings easily hurt?			
Are you very sensitive to hidden agendas or do you know what others are feeling even if they try to hide it?			
Do you have a wide range of emotions?			
Does your mood shift dramatically based on the people and events around you?			
Do you have a quick temper that also disappears quickly when the situation is no longer threatening?			
Are you physically sensitive to people or things?			
Are you soothed and/or aided in focusing by the use of a TV, radio, or fan?			
Are you empathetic?			
Do you have trouble getting places on time?			
Do you have difficulty determining how long a task will take?			

2

UNDERSTANDING YOURSELF

If you're interested in ADD as a diversity issue and wish to free yourself from an identity where you've been cast in the shadows of dysfunction into the light where you can be seen as the valuable person you are—one who is a commodity that benefits everyone and everything—this section is intended for you. You will learn to heal old wounds, begin your personal journey to find your *True Self*, and discover how to merge with a Linear world to which you will have learned to accommodate without further wounding.

The world needs you so it can become more balanced. Then your self-esteem and true identity will emerge to be valued as you share with others in order to bring a holistic approach to life for the good of all. No brainstyle can accomplish this job alone.

You are needed.
This Section is: For You

As many years ago as your age counts, there was a new being who came to live on this planet. You, the infant—filled with potential,

inspired to learn and grow, and vulnerable all at the same time—
began a journey.

How has your journey gone for you?
Consider how you feel about yourself and your life.
Now older, it's time to stop and assess how you are doing
on your journey.
Consider the following questions and decide how
you wish to continue:
Are you making the achievements you dreamed of making?
Or, do you feel lost?
What kind of road have you traveled?

No matter what your answers, you are valuable—whether you
feel that way or not. We'll begin to enrich your good feelings of
self, despite where you think your travels have taken you.

You passed through infancy and toddlerhood to learning to
play as a school-age kid, morphed into adolescence, and reached
young adulthood. Even if you're at a comfortable time in your
life, you may be concerned about the paths which your own adult
children or grandchildren are taking at this time. Or, it may be
your personal relationship with ADD that interests you as you
are approaching the growing-older adult stage of your life. At
this later time, you may even yearn to fill in any gaps that were
missed along the way.

Regardless of your age and stage in life, or feelings of success
or desperation, you are invited to walk with all of us to the healing
and happiness you deserve as you embrace your ADD.

Consider your desire to understand more about your brainstyle.
What unfinished business do you wish to take a look at?
Do you feel seriously wounded, empty, or incomplete?
Did you have wonderful dreams in your youth,
the fulfillment of which has eluded you?

The phrase, "If you can dream it, you can do it," though true, may infuriate you or trigger deep, heart-wrenching sadness and chronic depression or feelings of guilt as if you should have been able to achieve.

Your journey may be hard, but with new information and others who want to pass on what they have learned, you can come into your own and have a chance to reach your dreams. That's what this book is all about. It's *for you*—to embrace yourself, ADD and all.

THE FIVE STAGES FOLLOWING RECOGNITION OF OUR ADD

As often happens, we ADD folks recognize one another. We tend to think similarly, like similar things, share problems as we attempt certain activities, and laugh and cry at the same rewards and failures as we seek to come into our own. Though we each have unique variations that make us who we are, it seems that we go through the same stages of finding like kind when we come together in large groups.

There are five stages each of us goes through after we discover our ADD brainstyle, where we find others like us and begin to own ourselves with pleasure. Finally we come together to mentor others as we grow.

While mingling with over 300 participants at an early conference solely dedicated to serving adults with an ADD brainstyle in the early 1990s, the light bulb went off in my head. As it did, tears threatened to escape for all to see. I was viewing the happiness, healing, and growing of adults who previously had been lost or wanting, or whose lives were in disarray.

I recognized people with intense emotions: happiness, sadness, anger, excitement, euphoria, and peacefulness. These wonderful people were experiencing different levels of awareness and understanding about their ADD. I began to realize that what I was seeing were the stages through which we all go as we integrate information about our ADD brainstyle into our daily living. Five distinct stages emerged.

Stage One could be called the "Aha, I have it" stage. "Finally I have an explanation for why my life is the way it is. There really is something different about me. But I'm not crazy, mentally compromised, lazy, inadequate, or no good." This is a time of awakening. It's the recognition that "there are others like me." "I'm not the only one." Shock, excitement, and euphoria are likely to accompany this time along with an insatiable search for information.

Stage Two can be called the grief stage. Once the realization sinks in that there was a reason for not being able to live up to potential, the hurts, traumas, and losses suffered because of an ADD brainstyle begin to surface. As your mind begins to recall the hundreds of incidents that were related to ADD, your emotions begin to react. Confusion, anger, "what ifs," and depression all churn, creating emotional bedlam. This stage does end—but first it is important to feel your emotions thoroughly and grieve the losses in order to heal your wounds.

Stage Three could be called "the family stage" and involves seeking support and understanding companionship while grieving. Over and over at the Adult ADD Conferences, I heard people say, "I've found my family. There are others like me. I plan to come every year to my family reunion." Not only can information and guidance be gained at such groupings, but all-important emotional support can be obtained. "Coming home" to a place of unconditional acceptance heals the wounds of the past and supports the growth of the future.

Stage Four could be called the "growing up phase" and is characterized by seeking, exploration, and experimentation. It's a time for trying things. With ADD factored into a person's life, suddenly everything looks different. Exposure to previously tried experiences is necessary in order to discover from the new ADD perspective whether you like or dislike them, can or can't do them, want or don't want to pursue them now. It's an updating of data in one's bank of life experience that you want to continue to draw from.

Stage Five means coming of age. It is surely a time for the unfolding of a new identity. It's a time to redefine values, honor talents and gifts, and love who and what you are. "I know who I am now. I believe in myself. I can do whatever I've discovered I like. I am me." Reaching potential is wonderful, beautiful, and heady stuff. It is also possible and real.

LET'S GET STARTED ON THE WORK

The integration of current information into the life experiences of innumerable people is opening the door for the development of a valuable resource known to each of us: individual identity. As differences are recognized and honored, by yourself and others, not only will individual lives be made more pleasant, but the world will truly become a better place in which to live.

With this having been said, it's now time for us to take our first step to work together to assess and heal any wounding that happened, often inadvertently, during our developing life. Thanks to many who have gone before us, you will be able to take advantage of what they have learned. I will give you the gift of guidance. I ask from you in return that you give yourself honestly, to the best of your ability, to working on your own behalf. Then you can become a transmitter to those who follow you down this road.

If you and I were sitting down together and wanted to formalize this agreement between ourselves as we move forward into this journey of discovery and healing, here's what it would look like:

Our Working Agreement

My first gift to share with you is a way to sort through the time in your life that has preceded Now.

Your contribution is to consider what *fits* you, put aside what doesn't, and be scrupulously honest about your feelings. Under no conditions are you to judge yourself or others, or feel guilty about what you did or didn't do.

At this moment you have a fresh opportunity to fix what is not working for you by changing your behavior and strengthening what is right about you.

You are in charge, but you must make your choices honestly, based on your feelings and *not* on what others have said is the way to do things or the way to believe about yourself. Neither am I to tell you what is right or wrong. *Only you* know your truth, deep within yourself.

I will present you with options. You will have to decide which ones you want to pursue. I can inspire and encourage you, but only you can do the work.

I can listen to you as you speak of obstacles that you encounter. I can give you alternative solutions to try. I won't quit walking at your side until you reach the goal you wish to reach. At that time, the outcome belongs to you and will be reflected positively in your behavior and in your rising self-esteem as you begin to like yourself, as you become the person you were always meant to be.

Having gotten off track between birth and now—whether it is because of other people, your having failed because you were expected to do and be what didn't *fit* you, or because of woundings no matter what their origin—you can heal.

You can grow into your *True Self* and you can live the life that you've wanted to. Let's go for it!

Sign and Date _____

Think back to the times in your life that have contributed to the Current You. Step by step, you'll have the opportunity to reframe what happened that you want to change and recall the experiences that you want to keep. Maybe you will remember these experiences or recall stories told about you as a young child. See if there are photos of you taken during your first six early years. Look at that child with compassion, love, and acceptance even if it's hard to do. You can also shut your eyes and visualize any child of that age that you've seen or can imagine. Any of these ways will put you in touch with the young you. Even if the adult you feels like you're drawing a blank, your child part will feel you reaching out and will begin to reach back until you remember having connected.

Remember, you were an innocent child, one who confronted experiences that caused you to think you are less than you are capable of being.

In my journey while counseling and working with ADD, I've come in contact with four perspectives that have contributed to the way you are, affecting your growth and development and everyone else's for that matter. We'll discuss these in depth:

- The first is summed up by a general social-emotional theory of human nature, The Core Components of Human Nature (Weiss, 1976). It will lead you to ways to fix the wounding that may have compromised your well-being for much of your life.
- The second perspective focuses on the role played by family dysfunction and abuse in the home and other settings such as education (chapter 3, p. 81).
- The third looks at vulnerability to stress because of ADD attributes, sensitivity being one of the main culprits (chapter 3, p. 81).
- The fourth stems from the effects of sociocultural beliefs that cause wounding (chapter 3, p. 81).

THE CORE COMPONENTS OF HUMAN NATURE

The unfolding of the Core Components of Human Nature applies to all people in all cultures. It is a simple way of looking at a set of steps that lead us through the basics of how we grow socially and emotionally.

The five core components unfold naturally from birth to age six when each of us experiences a drive that causes us to:

- Develop a Sense of Trust that our needs will get met
- Manifest our Identity
- Develop a Sense of Competence
- Build a Sense of Powerfulness to get our own needs met
- Form a Sense of Self-Control that includes our ability to empathize with others and develop a conscience and a fledgling value system that stems from an internal desire to do what feels right within us.

From then on, we refine the components throughout our lives.

We Need What We Need When We Need It!

As we begin to explore the Core Components of Human Nature, we must remember that our human nature requires that each of us gets our needs met.

The trick is to get those needs met in socially acceptable, growth-producing ways that don't harm others or leave refuse and waste in their aftermath.

The stages of each component unfold automatically starting when we are born. How you are aided or thwarted in the development of each stage will greatly affect the remainder of your life.

The fact that you have an ADD brainstyle means that each of the five stages was affected by your Analogue nature. To enhance the social-emotional health of the core components, it is now useful to reinforce the development of ADD attributes and guard against further wounding because of ADD not being acknowledged as a diversity issue. As you continue to mature, you can remedy and strengthen the backbone of the social-emotional aspects of your well-being.

Because all young children are active, have short attention spans, and learn kinesthetically in the early years, one of the biggest gifts any child can be given is awareness and sensitivity to feel and express his or her needs. Hopefully you were not pushed as a preschooler to produce in traditional Linear ways.

The kids who fit a more Linear style of learning will let you know when they are ready to engage that aspect of themselves. The kids who have more Analogue attributes will not react well to pressure to move toward the Linear style of learning. If pressed to move toward a style of learning that does not *fit* them, they will begin the process of being wounded. They can learn the Linear system as a "second language," but it is very important during the first six years to support their Analogue system to avoid life-long hurt that stunts their development. Now let's talk about what we need to reinforce and heal.

What We Need to Reinforce and Heal:
The First Step

The First Core Component: A Sense of Trust
(Birth to Eighteen Months)

Here's what your first months would have looked like as you sought to learn to trust that you would get what you needed to feel safe and secure. Imagine yourself experiencing the following descriptions of what infancy might have been like for you.

"Mmmmm," comfortable, dry, not too hot or too cold, not hungry, feeling loved and played with, close to the ones who loved you. No worries.

But what if your mom was flighty and didn't get you fed on time? Maybe you were a "colicky" baby and had a lot of pain. Perhaps your dad was away and your mom was afraid she'd make mistakes, so she became very, very anxious—and you felt all that anxiety. Maybe Daddy's voice roared angrily and scared you. Or maybe your mom and dad fought a lot, partied a lot, and didn't pay much attention to you, so that comfort eluded you.

Not a very good way to build trust!

Sometimes no one meant to hurt you, but you got hurt nonetheless. Maybe you were like Jenny, a little girl whose skin was so sensitive that it made her squirm and lose sleep because the thread count of the sheets in her crib was not high enough to counteract the sensitivity of her skin. Her grandmother figured the problem out because she, too, had very sensitive skin. From then on, her parents carefully watched any cloth that came in contact with their daughter's skin. They also monitored the laundry soap and softeners for washing her clothes and were sure to use special soap for bathing.

Fortunately for Jennie, the problem was solved fairly readily and little long-term emotional hurt occurred. Whew!

Discomfort is the enemy of Trust building. Since infants can only cry to communicate to parents that something is wrong, parents become frustrated, feel helpless, and more stress builds as a result, compounding the situation.

Sensitivity is a key attribute for anyone with ADD and since it's genetic, it's likely to show up in multiple generations in the family. Check out your family history even if ADD was not identified. I'll bet you'll see attributes popping up here and there. Oh, and by the way, sensitivity is masked for many people beneath chemical dependency, anger, and rage problems.

Because this book is about a style of brain construction, you are likely to have other family members who have struggled, or are still struggling, with ADD—from grandparents to cousins and extended family members of all ages.

Hopefully, as you grew, your parents or caregivers got used to your communication and things worked better for you. Calmness and consistency would have been crucial to the building of Trust that your needs would get met. Too much change, such as moving, unsettles most babies so check out that part of your early history. Enough, but not too much touching, is good. On the other hand motion can drive many ADD babies wild, thus hurting their trust.

It's not always easy to tell whether a baby is going to turn out to have a large component of ADD attributes. One adult I knew started his early years with few signs of ADD. He was the easiest child in the world to attend to. In seconds, he fell asleep when rocked in his mother's arms. He was generally quiet, held long conversations as soon as he began to talk, and calmly went through early childhood. It seemed that he'd escaped ADD contributed by his dad's and mother's sides of the family.

In contrast, his brother was bothered by everything: eighteen-wheelers hurt his ears and new baby foods were spit out vigorously because there was simply too much new taste in his mouth at one time. SENSITIVITY reigned! And his activity level was definitely elevated beyond that of other preschoolers. But he was also very funny, outgoing, and active.

Other challenges to trust facing you during your first eighteen months included sound, music, and noise that was either too loud, too monotonous, or too overwhelming. Too much constant noise was felt in a hurtful manner. Being around arguing and fighting definitely would have disrupted the development of your Trust system.

ADD attributes made it hard for your Sense of Trust to develop. But if your family sensitively worked to shelter you and spared you too much damage to your developing emotional system, you would have come through without lasting damage. You ended up feeling at least moderately supported in your home. And you came out with an adequate level of Trust that your needs would get met. Great!

Look back at your experiences during your early life.
How were you affected by noise, skin sensitivity, rough play,
vacuum-cleaner noise, and such ADD stressors?

How did you fare? Tell your story orally or in writing.
Did you feel safe or was life scary?

Because ADD kiddos are likely to be more active and sensitive
than the average child, we may have been viewed as "problem
kids." High levels of action were likely as we grew up. It was up to
our families to learn to accommodate our special gift. With careful
protection, not too much and not too little, they would have been
able to help us retain our innate nature and build a Sense of Trust.

Look back at the complaints or stories about you, the baby.
What was said about you?
What didn't go so well for you?

A Sense of Trust is the most crucial of the five components,
utterly necessary for human emotions and socialization to develop
appropriately. It is hard to change if you didn't accumulate a reasonable amount of trust by age six. We all must continue to work
on our Sense of Trust throughout life, including the good, the bad,
and the ugly.

Though I don't expect you to believe me immediately, working
at connecting with your little inner kid to reassure him or her that
you'll be there is the most important way you can help yourself.
When needed, you can take little steps at first so you get used to
this kind of work. The little gal or guy within your memory banks
holds the key to the rest of your life.

Go slowly. That's much better than expecting results too soon
and ending up so disappointed that you quit. Take one step at a
time and celebrate with gratitude every positive gain you make, no
matter how small. Let go of others who tell you what you *should*
do, rather than suggesting what you *might* do. Spend time with
people who are working on their own growth. And, remember,
there are no "all grown up" people anywhere. Not anywhere.

Outcomes

Due to the development of a solid Sense of Trust, in adulthood you and your inner child will demonstrate the following signs of adequate Trust: security, patience, optimism, consistency, stick-to-itiveness, reliability, intimacy, and the ability to listen and to build interpersonal relationships.

Due to an underdeveloped Sense of Trust, you and your inner child will demonstrate the following signs of Low Trust: impulsivity, hoarding, suspiciousness, impatience, pessimism, trouble seeking help, difficulty with relations, and low risk-taking.

What We Need to Reinforce and Heal: The Second Step

The Second Core Component: Separation and Identity (Eighteen Months to Three Years)

At eighteen months to three years old, you began to encounter a new array of challenges as you started separating from your parent(s) or caregiver(s). At first, you probably ran a few steps away and began saying "No." Those were your beginning steps to becoming your own person. You were able to do that because you had gained enough trust to take those first tentative steps away from your zone of safety.

Your moves were designed to separate you from that source of everything you needed as a baby. Ah, but you were no longer a baby, were you? You became *You on wheels!*

But sadly, there are many adults who don't like to have children tell them "No." They think it's disrespectful and impolite. If this happened to you, instead of gaining a strong, healthy foundation for independence and self-esteem, you learned it wasn't safe to be you, to grow, achieve, and set boundaries.

The second mighty word during this period of separation and beginning identity formation would have been "Mine." Oh, how wonderfully selfish! "It's Mine!"

Unfortunately, many of us experienced scoldings and lectures about how we needed to share. But "no," the adults needed to learn that it's better to provide three cardboard boxes than one fancy store-bought toy for you and two of your friends to play with. Then, at two, you could have your very own cardboard box.

You, I, and all other kids were simply trying to figure out who we were by yelling out, "My doll!" Why don't adults get it? "I am what I possess" . . . at least at the age of two. Harsh socialization at this age that required you to prematurely share will more than likely have slowed down your ability be charitable with others at a later time.

Ironically, the more you, the child, were validated with, "That's right, the doll is your doll," the more you learned to share easily at age three and beyond. Giving a sibling or visitor another doll or toy to play with contributed to your becoming an adult who tends to be generous and able to let go to share with others later in life.

Later, when you had to deal with learning attributes that didn't *fit* you, you likely found it hard to stand up for what was right for *you*. You may have given way to politeness, been too good, and failed to protect your wonderful inner *True Self*. If that's the case, you'll need to help the two-year-old part of you to learn to be independent. You can do it.

Recall your own experiences with sharing.
Were you scolded for not sharing?
Does your family recall sharing being a problem for you?

I'd like to share with you the treatment of wounding with reframing (relearning.) This skill will be used throughout the book and can become a tool that you use with the part of you that has suffered wounding at an earlier time in your life.

I want to tell you about an eight-year-old ADD child who had trouble sharing. His teacher sighed as she asked me to help her deal with the child by saying, "He's restless, has trouble maintaining a focus on his desk work, and acts like a two-year-old." As I watched him, I immediately saw that he harbored a two-year-old within who had probably been forced to over-share as a little boy.

The teacher began to help him in a kindly way to learn as if he were two. She did not in any way embarrass or shame him in the process. She simply reinforced his "his-ness" with his schoolwork, possessions, and relationships. She commented, "You are a good friend the way you share your pencils." "This week you took your turn in line at the lunchroom, so I'd like you to be the line leader next week." You should have seen the broad grin on his face when he heard that.

Interestingly, as he was helped to progress by dealing with his two-year-old needs, he began to settle down and pay better attention in class. His identity was able to grow beyond the original age where it had gotten stuck. Then the rest of his maturation could tag along, slowly helping him focus on more age-appropriate behavior despite his ADD. By the end of the year, he'd caught up with the other kids in class. By then he knew how to share. And he could better articulate what he needed to learn in his special ADD way. He could say, "I need it to be quiet to read." Not only did he know what he needed but he felt worthy to ask for it.

Another factor to consider at the eighteen month to three-year-old stage is that little ones are kinesthetic learners. Actually, each of us was a kinesthetic learner from birth, but it wasn't as apparent during the first eighteen months because the child was less mobile. At this second stage, is it ever apparent! It can be a major contributor to wounding that most children face.

Think of it this way. Any bright kid who is curious—and was not likely to "hang out" quietly with their mom and dad, grandparents, or anyone else, sitting sedately on a blanket in the park—felt a lot of pressure to sit still. It's as if she's saying, "I need to touch 'it,' the grass, feel 'them,' the rocks, and play with anything with which I come in contact, including the silverware in the restaurants."

But being an ADD kid means the effects of your kinesthetic nature extend for a lifetime. It was to my chagrin that I patted the belly of a bronze statue of a toddler at the Dallas Museum of Art when I was attempting to introduce some artistic culture to my school-age boys.

Imagine their faces and my embarrassment when the gallery guard suddenly appeared, scowled, and said, "Ma'am, do not touch the sculpture." I immediately looked around to see who might have noticed my faux pas. Alas, besides guilt, I felt cheated from the joy of a hands-on viewing of such a beautiful art work. Thus speaketh a seriously kinesthetic ADD adult.

Can you relate to this?
If so, have a laugh and know we're all in good company.

Maybe our motto for Linear learning ought to be "hands-off" learning, not "hands-on learning."

Oh well, there's really not that much wrong with being so full of touch. But it's hard not to grow up thinking we are irresponsible or have "behavior problems" when we were continually told, "Don't touch that." "What's the matter with you? Keep your hands to yourself." "I can't take you anywhere without your getting in trouble." Such rebuffs and scoldings were bad for your self-esteem.

Ironically, it wasn't any better for me. I never got into trouble. I was the perfect "only" child of older parents. They could be heard saying with a big smile when telling their friends, "We can take her anywhere. She behaves better than most adults. We're so proud of her."

I recall feeling uncomfortable when all eyes fell upon me. I didn't know why. In retrospect, I suspect that somehow I knew this state of affairs wasn't normal—whatever that meant to a child. All I knew was that I seemed to know how to get along with adults but didn't have a clue about relating to other children, which meant getting into trouble.

True, I wasn't getting into trouble like the other kids, but I sure wasn't happy. I was sad and felt guilty a lot of the time because I wanted to touch everything. I felt deprived. I was as curious and eager to investigate everything as any healthy child would have been. But I held back, sat straight, and felt tense, despite being a strongly kinesthetic child. Wow, have I changed in seven decades!

Growing up, I'll bet that you, like me, could almost feel the grass growing beneath you. Likely you would have urgently felt the need to run—an urgency that you only now can put into words. "I, too, felt I *had* to run around in a circle, jump up on anything that extended in the air, and roll through the leaves in the fall." Our urges were a response to the questions pulsing through our bodies. "How far can I go on my two fast legs? How high can I jump? How much can I roll? What does all of this action feel like? I want it."

Sure, you may vaguely have heard someone calling you to come back, but there's no way you were going to be able to give up your newfound freedom of motion and independence, if you felt safe to go against the people who were raising you. So you didn't turn back.

Hopefully, you experienced age-appropriate guidance through this period—guidance that was free of punishment and threats. Guidance that set up safety guidelines and simple, sensible limits with lots of opportunities to follow the urgings of childhood yearnings. Logical consequences and simple time-outs are enough behavioral direction for preschoolers.

With the onset of age three, a gift awaited you if you were supported and strengthened as a two-year-old with a budding sense of self and the ability to recognize who you were becoming. Healthy development of your early identity had a hidden treasure contained within it for you, if you had been neither seriously abused nor neglected.

The gift was a fledgling identity that automatically reflected high self-esteem and awareness of how special you were and would be.

If you were neglected or over-punished, high self-esteem may have failed to appear during this open window of time. You can work on it as an adult and, though you're playing catch-up, you'll be in a position to live a better life than you ever imagined.

Outcomes

Due to the development of solid Self-Awareness, you and your inner child will demonstrate the following signs of high adequacy: Independence, individuality, leadership, ease of sharing, clear self-awareness, the ability to set goals and make decisions, the ability to play clear roles and serve specific purposes.

Due to an underdeveloped Self-Awareness, you and your inner child will demonstrate the following signs of low adequacy: Dependency, vacillation, indecision, possessiveness, and lack of leadership, clarity of opinions, interests, or purposes.

What We Need to Reinforce and Heal: The Third Step

The Third Core Component: A Sense of Competence (Three Years to Four Years)

The age of three to four is naturally meant to be a great time to be living. Originally you felt good about yourself when the third core component surfaced at about thirty-six months. With it came the wonderful gift of feeling that it is supported by being able to count on getting your basic needs met and enjoying an identity that is *yours, all yours!*

Of course, you are going to feel as if you can do all sorts of things. You feel competent. Three to four is the time that you believe, "I can do it!" You're experiencing an innate sense of competence. "I can do *anything!*"

Next let's sprinkle in a curious, inventive, aspiring, active ADD mind and body to the mix. Camera! Action!

If you had the space to run around, enough play opportunities, and a semi-structured day to begin to get used to a little structure, you had the basic resources to draw upon for your feelings of competence to grow. You would have wanted to do everything that you saw the adults doing.

Unfortunately, your inner urges were bigger and stronger than your ability to actually reach a goal of doing "them." This early Sense of Competence is only a feeling, a sense. Granted it will morph into high-level skills as an adult, but at age three, your cognitive perception of doing things was quite poor—so you didn't really see ahead of time or experience what the outcome might look like. At three, it was all about the process of doing, rather than about the achievement of a goal or end result.

Thus you might have believed you could pour your own milk from a gallon jug into your small child's glass. And your belief would have been strong enough to go for it without even being shown how to do it. Odds are you either dropped the six-plus pound milk carton on the floor or missed the little glass, spilling milk all over the table and floor.

But, you wouldn't really have minded because you felt you knew how to clean up such spills. Ah, one more activity to feel good about. You'd seen your mom or dad clean spills up. So you'd get out the towel and water and slosh the milk and water over a large space on the floor before putting the wet mopping rags into the dryer—possibly on top of a batch of clean clothes. Well, aren't dryers for drying?

From your perspective, the job was well done. From your parent's perspective, "What a mess!"

Wise parents provided small child-sized pitchers to pour from and supervised the "doing" of all the wonderful things that you wanted to do. But oh, my, it takes patience to work with a three-year-old. It also takes twice as long when children help. It also means that your accomplishments were less than well done, but that never was the point. It was all about the process.

Remember, process and function are strong suits for ADD people, much more than the details of whatever you're doing, thinking, or dreaming about.

What's your story?
How did your trying and "doing" work turn out for you?

If you were scolded or left alone to get into unsupervised trouble, barked at for "messing everything up," told "Can't you do anything right?" then your fragile gift of confidence would have evaporated quickly, replaced by fears of making mistakes.

If you had a perfectionistic parent or relative around who did all the things you yearned to do, your confidence also could have gotten compromised. Or worse yet, you might have been banished from the workroom with no return offered. Perfectionism and a three-year-old don't mix well. That dreadful fear of making mistakes would have grown, haunting you even today, as an adult. Better you learned to inhibit what you did, reign in your ADD desire to try new things, experiment, and experience broadly than risk the fear and humiliation of doing things that were wrong.

Likely as an adult, you'll blame yourself for being clumsy and mistake-prone. You may even ride your own case incessantly trying endlessly to get things right. Lots of your fellow ADD companions will be suffering like you, but feel too embarrassed to let you know.

Or the opposite: Do you apologize endlessly about making any mistakes, warning everyone that you are inept, never could do "it," and go on and on as a recording of stress and tension? Ironically, stress raises the odds of creating a mistake—it is a setup for failure.

Were you stressed by living with perfectionism
or a serious taskmaster?

Did you feel humiliated because you couldn't do something that
a younger sibling or friend could do?

You need to realize there are so many things to learn that there
is no good way to choose which ones to practice now that you're
an adult.

You must realize that everyone is different. Maybe you can run
fast and so could your little kid. Maybe she absolutely loved water,
kicking, splashing, and learning to dive. It may not have gotten
you to the Olympics but oh, you loved it. Or maybe you were not
physically inclined, but you loved building things and working with
your hands (small motor coordination). Or maybe you talked—a
lot. You say, "What's so special about talking?" Well, I'll tell you.
It makes friends, entertains people, and helps you teach others,
even at three.

So, I ask you,
What is one special skill you've always had?
Do not laugh at it or discount it. That would be
repeating how someone else looked at it.
Your job is to tell your little kid, "Wow, you
do _____ really well. You're super."
Go ahead and hug the little kid in your mind.

Wild and Neglected

If you were allowed to be wild, or neglected, left alone too
much, you may not have received some timely early training in
your "second language" that would have gently prepared you for
the Linear world you would be entering in kindergarten.

Age three was a wonderful time to have begun to be taught
the ways of the alien world of Linear living, an efficient, fun time
to begin learning the process of doing things. To whatever degree

you weren't taught skills that are a normal part of adult living, step up to your little one within and start the process now. I don't care how inept you feel you are. You *can* do it, one step at a time. And, your inner kid sure can learn plenty from you. If you find a teacher other than yourself, be cautious to find a noncritical, brainstyle-balanced teacher from whom you can learn without being wounded. A great starting point is to begin to teach yourself how to put away things in their "home."

Making Mistakes

If mistakes have haunted you, here's a training regime for you. One of the biggest problems facing all children after age three is their fear of making mistakes. Add to that the additional tendency of Analogue young ones to work fast, be especially inquisitive, and be emotionally eager to do something that feels awesome.

Oh, how exciting to see the end product in one's mind! But, how difficult to not naturally know the steps that lead to success in reaching the end vision. What a setup for mistakes and disappointment. Thus lots of examples of anxiety and fear have usually been accumulated by the time a child reaches the teen and adult years.

Try This: Make a Mistake a Day!

Start by purposely making one mistake a day and then fix it up. I don't care which one you pick. Anything will do. Then tell yourself, "Hey, great, little one." You gave you and your kid a learning opportunity. Thank you. You got to fix up the mistake, which will make your day.

When you fix up a pesky mistake, get ready to celebrate. Choose something, before you start, to use for your treat, something healthy that you and your kid really like. You have to choose your treat now, because together you can't fail.

You will notice soon that your little kid's fear level about making mistakes will begin to decline—so that your adult self either becomes less irritable and angry or less nervous and anxious. Either way, you win. Then you qualify to be a regular, fallible human being with all the rest of us. Welcome to the world of imperfection!

When someone says you were clumsy or accident-prone, remember that you are someone who loves to do things. You may be making more mistakes than your Linear counterparts. But, percentage-wise you'll be making fewer mistakes because you are trying to do so many more things.

The Story of Three-Year-Old Budding Engineers

In the 1990s, I was talking with two mothers in a child-development training class about the three Es of a Sense of Competence: Experience, Experiment, and Expression. It seems that each of them had raised a son who, at the time of the class, was in his thirties. One mom frowned, still looking stressed, when she recalled the problems she encountered when her son was three years old.

"It seems that all he did was mess up the house. I spent all my time cleaning and straightening," she said. "We bought him all kinds of games and toys, but he didn't want to play with them. He just wanted to take things apart, stir things up, and go through the trash. He took the knobs off the radio and TV but wouldn't put them back on, he would fill a bowl with whatever he could find and haul out my mixer so he could make 'soup' pretending he was a chef.

"One day I found all the tools from his father's tool box strewn around the house. I could tell he had been trying to figure out how to use them on everything and anything he could reach, indoors and outdoors. You should have seen the scratches and broken pieces of wood and nails everywhere! Not a single thing had been put back together. Nothing was put back where he'd gotten it.

"I scolded him good, gave him a spanking, and put locks on all the cupboards and doors where I kept things. I made him stay in his play room with all those nice toys. On sunny days he could play outside on the jungle gym."

The second mom had been chuckling and nodding her head throughout most of the story. It seems her son also wanted to take everything apart. He tried to stick things in the electric outlets and build with scraps of wood he found using nails and a hammer from the woodshed.

Her solution was a bit different, however. She decided to join him when she could to "make" things, gave him a place to put his "found" objects, and then they had a snack "party" after clean-up time.

Together they went around the house and put red stickers on the things that he must not touch and green stickers on cabinets that he could take the knobs off of. He could also clear out the pots and pans drawer and use the garden tools. He had his own stash of nails and a hammer. She let him show off what he'd made to his dad after work, even if it was a piece of wood with one streak of paint on it. And, fortunately, dad paid attention and everyone clapped.

This mom said her house wasn't fit for company for a few years. But as time went on, her son learned to put back together what he'd taken apart, became a "fix-it boy" as an older child, and eventually became an engineer as an adult—an adult who loved playing "grown-up kid" and making good money as a professional.

The child in the first story never found a job or career that he really liked and he struggled with his Sense of Competence throughout his life. He tried maintenance work, but it wasn't challenging enough. He thought about becoming an engineer, but he was too fearful to try to go for the degree.

His mom wasn't a "bad" mom. She simply didn't know or sense that he was a kinesthetic learner who needed to Experience, Experiment, and Express his way through the stage when he took things apart—before a later stage when he would learn to put things together. Nor did she realize that he, like all three-year-olds, needed guidance to begin to learn simple organizational skills that would help guide him. She didn't know how to channel his innate skills.

I ask you to look back at your three-year-old period.
Remember the stories that were told about you: "Oh no" stories about all the "really awful things you did," or the stories that were told with humor about the "things you got into."
Now, I suggest you work with your own inner three-year-old.
What is *your* story with Experiencing, Experimenting, and Expressing?
Next, figure out about what age you need to start with.
Talk or write about an incident that pops in your mind.
Do you have a three-year-old within you who needs to mess?
Or do you know how to use some tools, but not well?
Do your hands tingle at the thought of becoming skillful with tools?
How about taking a class?
You may just find the "parent-teacher" you didn't have.
And you will grow and grow with confidence as you truly "learn more things."
Or is your inner child a young girl or boy who simply needs to immerse yourself in a "hobby" that could even become a job or profession with some more training?
Let yourself explore.
Keep your day job if you need the money, but go ahead and immerse yourself in this new learning.
It can turn the light up bright in your heart and soul.

I certainly understand this issue on a personal level. After retiring from the peak of my clinical career, I took two years to explore becoming a professional artisan. I'd been doing arts and crafts since I was five years old and nearly chose art as my initial major in college. Instead, I chose a different path but never stopped wondering whether I might still want to manifest that part of my dream.

As it turned out, I decided I'd prefer to keep art as a joyful avocation. It was a relief, however, to no longer wonder what I might have been able to do and whether I could have been competent at doing art. It turned out to be more work than I wanted to put into it. And I really only wanted to design one thing one time and then switch to creating something totally different. How ADD! That's just fine. My heart is more committed to writing and dialoguing with others. I can play with my art as a wonderful outlet. I'm glad I found this out.

Outcomes

Due to the development of a solid Sense of Competence, you and your inner child will demonstrate the following signs of high adequacy: Expressiveness, curiosity, willingness to try new things, ability to recoup from mistakes and failures, a unique perspective on a job, self-motivation, ability to ask questions, and the ability to be creative.

Due to an underdeveloped Sense of Competence, you and your inner child will demonstrate the following signs of low adequacy: Say "I can't," hide mistakes, procrastinate indefinitely, demonstrate perfectionism, experience embarrassment in taking credit for a good job, inhibit expressiveness, fear being asked questions, and avoid learning situations.

What We Need to Reinforce and Heal: The Fourth Step

The Fourth Core Component: A Sense of Powerfulness (Four to Five or Five-and-a-Half Years)

"BAAAT MAAAN!" you sang and yelled at the top of your lungs as down you swooped off the dining-room table. That's you at four years old. Oh, what a wonderful feeling. So strong, so powerful, so SO! Well, that was until you heard your mom's feet coming toward you. And, sure enough, she enters the room with a frown on her forehead. And out of her mouth came the dreaded words, "What am I going to do with you? You were such a nice three-year-old."

You didn't want to disappoint your mom or have her get mad. You just wanted to show her how big and strong you'd become. You thought she'd be proud of you.

You didn't want to be "not nice." And you didn't know what happened to you. You didn't plan any of this. You sure didn't know "it" was coming. But suddenly it seemed that everything you used to like a few weeks earlier didn't seem important any more. You no longer wanted to help out around the house. You wanted to go way down the street, farther than you'd ever gone before, to places your dad said you couldn't go. "Son," he'd say, "You may only go two houses on either side of our house."

"That's NOT ENOUGH!" you thought but didn't say. "Maybe," you thought, "I'll just go when he's at work."

Ah, the story of a four-year-old who's learning to manipulate situations to get what he wants because his social-emotional job is to develop a Sense of Powerfulness to get his OWN needs met. No more waiting around for others to meet his needs.

After all, you trusted that others would get you what you need, you have separated from your mom and dad and know who you are becoming. You feel moderately competent to do anything that you want to do and believe you can get the job done yourself. It feels like the time to be really independent and important.

Do you remember that time?
Super Heroes, racing way down the street, running out of sight of your mom to have a tea party by the pond, or being able to argue with anyone about anything, including your parents and older siblings?

Despite your intent, you probably got into more trouble once you turned four than at any time earlier in your life. The worst part about it was that you didn't even know what you were doing wrong. You were just trying to be in charge of what you needed—or thought you needed.

Unless your parents were sensibly relaxed about your behavior, you more than likely were told many times "don't do that," or were put on time-out, or, worse yet, felt the wrath of their anger upon you.

What you needed to know was how to be powerful at the same time that you stayed safe and within acceptable boundaries, so neither you nor anyone or anything else got hurt. This stage of social-emotional development is the most complicated of the five stages. You need to be able to get your own needs met within the reasonable limits and boundaries set by the adults who were responsible for you.

So the wise parent, seeing you leap off the tall table yelling "BAAAT MAAAN!" needed to say to you, "Wow, look how big and strong and powerful you are." And then she needed to add, quickly and firmly, "But tables aren't for standing on. I do want to see you climb and be high up in the air and see how strong you are. Come on, let's go to the backyard. You can get up on the wall (or climbing gym, or . . .). Anytime you want me to see how strong you are, come find me, and I'll watch you jump off anything that is safe."

Later, confident that you understood about limits in your new extended world, she might have said, if she were a really smart mom, "Say, how would you like to make a deal with me about going to your friend's house five houses down the street? I see how responsible you are becoming, so I think you're ready. What you have to do is tell me where you want to go so I know where I can find you. Deal?"

"Deal!" you undoubtedly shouted.

"Oh, and if you forget to tell me, you'll need to stay inside the next day. Got it?"

Limit set—and that's why she was smart.

You knew a good thing when you heard it. "I won't forget."

She's got you right where she wanted you, because she had two things you really wanted: freedom and power.

"Okay," Mom says. Then mom keeps a sharp eye on you for a while to be sure you're ready to be trustworthy. If you aren't able to stay within the agreed-upon limits, she will need to reel you in rather than punish you. It would only mean the limits need to be narrowed for a while until you're ready for them to again be adjusted for size.

How did it go for you?
Were you taught how to respect limits
as you extended your powerfulness?
Did you understand boundaries?
Did you get good guidance in the expansion of your limits?
or
Were you left on your own with no guidelines so that you got
in trouble by discovering after the fact that what you did
was looked upon with disapproval?
What happened then?
Did you get yelled at? Or punished physically?

If you were threatened a lot, physically and emotionally punished, or overly constricted from expressing your budding powerfulness, your Sense of Powerfulness probably lagged behind, and the guidelines created by limits and boundaries failed to become strong for you at that time. It means that you were trying to behave yourself without proper training to do a good job.

You may have become an adult with a low Sense of Powerfulness despite the amount of status or authority you hold. You may suffer from anxiety or depression or perhaps you use brute force rather than discussion to attempt to settle things—all this because things didn't go very well when you were a four-year-old kid.

Add to that the frustration of being wounded because of your style of brain construction and you may be emotionally suffering now. When you couldn't use the innate intelligence that you have because of the way in which you learn things, you probably felt inadequate and helpless to do anything to change it. If you could do a job, but couldn't keep track of the paper work, you undoubtedly felt frustrated. In time your self-esteem would get tarnished, and that's a recipe for depression or blaming behavior. If you are unable to keep a nice house so that your really great husband can bring business friends over for dinner, you may feel seriously guilty and worthless.

Symptoms of low powerfulness in adults include telling lies, even "white" ones, failing to pursue goals in a way that fits your brainstyle, manipulating others, and being overly aggressive with temper outbursts, blaming behavior, and hidden feelings of vulnerability. Paranoia is a key attribute of low emotional powerfulness.

It's hard to trust a person with low power because that person has to self-protect because of the fear they feel that their needs won't get met.

Sadly, the behavior is passed from generation to generation when a parent, low in powerfulness, fails to have the ability to teach their children a way to break the cycle through action and modeling.

If this sounds like your deepest buried secret, you may have feelings of rage or its opposite, hopelessness and deep depression. And this might have been going on since childhood. It's all about not having found ways to get what you need for yourself and not having received what you needed from others.

But regardless of your parents' behavior, when a Linear belief system says, "We're the best, the acceptable, the desired way to be," and "You're disordered," your Sense of Powerfulness as an ADD person will be reduced. You've not only been abused, but you are likely to feel that there is something deeply wrong with you, rather than feeling as if the abuse is coming from outside of you. The only "power" you have is to believe that you are at fault. That way you carry hope that you can fix that awful, cloying feeling of wrongness.

Our culture hasn't evolved to the development of a high Sense of Powerfulness. So ADD is diagnosed and labeled while you are blamed and seen in an inferior way. A sign of Powerfulness means that a person or group takes the responsibility to get its own needs met, but not at anyone else's expense. Labeling takes worth away from you by pathological judgments that reduce your value.

Winning and losing are a part of building a strong Sense of Self-Control—with the person being powerful but not *over* anyone else. Everyone must win or be less than.

Abuse from outside of the immediate family might also lay down a foundation for low powerfulness and victimization. The innate sensitivity of being an Analogue person means that many experiences on the playground or in the classroom, neighborhood, and workplace are hurtfully felt. These settings provide fertile environments for the loss of power, often unseen by parents, teachers, bosses, or other adults.

The result may have set you up to lose your natural power—power that everyone needs to live a secure, fruitful life. Like a garden full of variegated plants and animals living in their natural habitats, everyone must be seen as valuable, only different. That is the way Diversity operates in nature. That is what Brainstyle Diversity is all about.

If reading any of this makes you uncomfortable, you can be pretty sure that your early path led you to need to work on emotional power building now. Most of us Analogue folks need to do this even coming from the best, much less worst, of parenting styles. The inequity caused by growing up in cultures with values and beliefs that don't support Analogue skills easily leads to a Sense of Low Powerfulness.

None of us gets through all five Core Components of Human Nature unblemished. We get off track, fail to develop in certain areas, and yet end up fairly okay. But because our ADD is so inextricably intertwined with our emotional experiences, we will need to help the child part within each of us heal any wounding that is holding us back. It takes courage and belief in ourselves to find and develop our *True Selves*.

Build your power one step at a time by telling the truth and supporting those who are needier and weaker than you. Ask for help. And, oh yes, don't forget to protect and support the parts of yourself that are vulnerable. You can do it!

Outcomes

Due to the development of a solid Sense of Powerfulness, you and your inner child will demonstrate the following signs of high adequacy: Ability to be responsible; ability to state what is wanted; assertiveness, not aggression; ability to say "No!"; willingness to win, but the ability to lose gracefully; willingness to be a follower, not only a leader; good judgment and follow-through; appropriate defense of self and others; effective management; implementation of goals, ideas, and dreams into action.

Due to an underdeveloped Sense of Powerfulness, you and your inner child will demonstrate the following signs of low adequacy: Acting irresponsibly; feeling overwhelmed, aggressive, and continuously furious; bullying; inability to say "No!"; acting wishy-washy; telling lies; working only on behalf of the underdog.

What We Need to Reinforce and Heal: The Fifth Step

The Fifth Core Component: A Sense of Self-Control (Five to Six-Plus Years)

As you work on your adult Sense of Powerfulness, you will be able to move toward control of yourself more and more. It is sort of like being able to count on yourself to do what you need and want day by day. Your courage will then lead you to the fifth and final step in achieving Self-Control.

Acting and thinking for yourself: The first four Core Components of Human Nature lead us to become responsible, motivated, and trustworthy with a firm grasp of our identity. With our foundation in place, we can be counted on to begin to control ourselves, rather than being controlled by threats, guilt, or force. Ultimately, we each want to do what is right for ourselves and in relation to others.

All of us get some degree of the social-emotional skills that we need in order to develop Self-Control: A Sense of Trust, an Identity, a Sense of Competence, and a Sense of Powerfulness. But we may also have to work to overcome some wounding that leads us to do what we *should* do instead of what we *want* to do. In order to get beyond the language of *shoulds* and *ought tos,* we need to do what we do because we consciously *choose* to do it for ourselves.

How do you learn what's right for you? By age five, many different things had already happened to you leading to the development of your first values and the development of a fledgling conscience. First of all, the value system you began to acquire is going to be the one with which you were raised.

You will also begin to develop empathy—empathy being the ability to feel what others are feeling. It's different from the sympathy that you've felt for another person. You may even identify with another's experience and feel sympathy. But to have empathy, your ability to feel the same way as another—whether you've had the experience or not—has to be functioning if you are to become self-controlled.

I think of it as "catching" feelings as opposed to "knowing about" what happened.

Empathy doesn't seem to occur before age five. It is totally dependent upon your having developed a Sense of Trust the first eighteen months followed by three-and-a-half more years of learning experience to trust that your needs will continue to be met.

From the growth of empathy, your conscience will begin to surface. It makes you want to follow the values with which you've been surrounded. And it makes you feel guilty when you don't. This, then provides a foundation for Self-Control. You try to act with right behavior because you feel good when you do, instead of becoming fearful of the repercussions of not doing so or because you want the approval of the important people in your life. It's not about outside constraints and approval. It's about inner control because of your beliefs.

Sure, you don't want negative consequences for not following rules. You also still like approval. But there's something else operating. You—the you who's been growing since age two—wants to do what's right because you *want* to.

Hopefully, you had a moderately supportive upbringing so the building blocks of Self-Control are at least fairly strong. I wish that for everyone. But if your parents or caregivers did not fare so well, you probably didn't either.

Unhealthy and nonconstructive parenting behaviors would raise the odds of your having a tough road to walk to achieve strong and healthy Self-Control. Sometimes the culture in which you were raised also had beliefs that worked against a healthy development of Self-Control. And maybe you and your family faced devastating conditions beyond everyone's control because of natural disasters, wars, financial or social unrest, or health issues.

What was, and is, the culture like in which you grew up?
How do you feel it shaped your beliefs and values?
How much room has there been for diversity to be practiced,
especially in relation to your brainstyle?
What challenges have you faced because you are an
Analogue processor?

No matter how the child part of you was trained, we can work together with many others around the world to repair weak and wounded Self-Control in those of us who have been less fortunate.

After childhood gives way to adolescence, you will have emerged into a time of questioning your family's values—the values with which you were raised. It's a time to experiment with which family values you want to keep and which ones you want to change to fit how you are thinking and feeling. Often this process continues through your twenties or even thirties or longer. Becoming a spouse and parent also tends to influence the mature values that you settle on. Not infrequently, young couples return to the value systems with which they were raised.

Sometimes it takes much of one's lifetime to sort through how you wish to believe. One young woman described the process this way. "I felt like a 'package of learned behaviors.' I didn't like the way it made me feel so I asked myself, 'Where is my heart, my soul, and the *True Me*?'" No wonder she spent much of her professional life seeking to find herself and Self-Control.

And, indeed, she became a psychotherapist who continually learned about herself while performing her professional role of helping others find themselves. She never stopped questioning her values, but consistently strengthened her Self-Control by eliminating "should" and "ought tos" from her behavioral choices.

Look at your extended family's history.
Check out the elements that make up your Self-Control:

The value system you were taught;
What you believe now, including the *shoulds;*
The fear you lived with because you were afraid
not to do what you were taught?
Are you accepting of different beliefs others choose to
live by without trying to change them to be like you?
Are you responsible for your actions by being self-monitoring,
reliable, predictable, empathetic, and accepting of help—or do
you have to work to maintain these virtues?
Have you faced devastating conditions: wars, natural disasters,
financial ruin, or overwhelming health or loss challenges?
Write or talk about how this affected you
and your immediate family.
If you feel considerable emotional stress, connect with
a spiritual or psychological professional counselor to
help you through your challenge.

Outcomes

Due to the development of a solid Sense of Self-Control, you and your inner child will demonstrate the following signs of high adequacy: Reliability; predictability; responsibility for your actions and the ability to self-monitor; good judgment; empathy and playfulness; strong morals; ability to accept help when needed; ability to act in ways that you personally believe in (the *wants*) rather than the way someone else says you should act (the *shoulds*).

Due to the underdevelopment of a Sense of Self-Control, you and your inner child will demonstrate the following signs of low adequacy: Losing control under the influence of drugs, alcohol, sex, and peer or work pressure; exhibiting impatience; inability to play; always needing to be in control; inability to accept help when needed; acting based on *shoulds* rather than on *wants;* acting out of guilt; and acting intolerant of differences.

And normal, adolescent growth and rebellion is a lot about defining one's values. During this time of chaos, many young people "find themselves." For you, it means you can begin to embrace your ADD.

Finding yourself as you look at the world in a way that is different from the norm isn't easy, as you know. Nor does the journey always look pretty. Lots of trial and error may be involved. This also means making many mistakes from which you can learn. Such mistakes can be turned into a benefit if, indeed, you figure out what you did wrong. Then you can do your personal healing and avoid taking the same faulty tracks leading to your future.

With a positive diversity approach to your Analogue processing brainstyle, you can become your own best friend and supporter. You can believe that your way is the best way for you. You can commit to healing previous wounding while learning new Analogue ways to function effectively with strength and success on your journey to Self-Appreciation and Achievement of the kind you value.

Henry Tells His Story: "I'm Not a Label, but a Work In Progress"—A Story of Self-Control Late in the Making, But Worth Waiting For

Part I: Henry, The Kid

At first blush, there didn't seem to be much ADD wounding showing up in Henry's childhood history. Rather shy early on and not a troublemaker according to parents and teachers, he was a typical only child who got along well with adults.

He, like all the rest of the kindergartners, was a kinesthetic learner, so he *fit* in fine—for a while. Trial-and-error learning was his best friend even into high school physics class experiments. Hands-on learning continued to be the name of his game.

When he was learning to read, it was slow going. He found it difficult until he got a tutor. Having a person present to encourage him even with the first tiny steps made all the difference. The tutor also gave him tools that helped him break down the reading process. As an adult, Henry credits his tutor's gift of reading tools for his learning to get past his reading "problem."

In general, book learning didn't work for Henry. Obviously smart, he would get math problems right by doing them in his own way, free of having been taught the "right" way and in a manner that was different than either the teacher or the book showed how to do them.

By middle school he was no longer engaged in his work except when he had a teacher with a personality that was challenging and empathetic and who picked up on emotions. The personal touch made him want to do better, and he would. Otherwise, he'd spend his time debating with his teacher. His grades went from "A"s to "C"s to failing.

His mom tells how Henry as a child would circle around the walls of a room before interacting with anyone, be it another child or an adult. Henry continued to be initially nervous about interacting with peers throughout school so that it took him a long time to get involved.

Two things brought him out of his shell: sports and his interest in creating his own businesses. The first of several business ventures started in high school and he continued to try new ideas after he graduated from high school and began part-time college studies. Henry's restless energy found a place to be discharged as he thought about a new business and turned it into a money-making venture. Entrepreneurship served him well.

He describes his late teens and early twenties as times to experiment, trying to find what he wanted to do, and figuring out who he wanted to be. It also was a time to learn to put on psychological armor when he was around others.

In looking back at the early history of Henry's life, you'll notice that his choices reflected potential ADD traits that could, and did, stay with him into adulthood. Some of them have served him well—and others left him without skills that caused wounding later.

At first, it seemed he was home free of ADD-related difficulties. But all that happened is that he dodged a bullet that was attached to a boomerang. His intelligence and ability to create his own way of going about accomplishing tasks left him without the drudgery of Linear skill-building. But later, when he really needed some experience with structure and discipline, he didn't have it and paid a high price for the deficit.

Let's take a look at key ADD attributes and styles that have followed Henry into adulthood. Each are typical attributes shared by various ADD adults.

Henry's ADD Makeup

Talking at length with Henry, it became apparent that, while a shy child who did not race around with a great deal of apparent hyperactivity, he was very active mentally. And, as he moved into his teen years, his ADD showed itself through multiple entrepreneurial enterprises. He was constantly involved in thinking about ways to create money, selling a product, and developing small businesses from yard work to delivery services.

Though he learned to be a good salesperson, basically he remained shy, not letting others really know him. He didn't let anyone see his vulnerability or feelings. Most of his interactions were business related, not personal, and did not allow him much of a private life.

Henry, the Kinesthetic Learner

As we said earlier, young children are primarily kinesthetic and hands-on learners. They have to touch everything first with their mouths and then with their hands. We can't tell at this early age whether a person is ADD or not.

When trial-and-error learning continued as the preferred mode of learning into middle and high school, it verified the style that belonged to Henry. The liking for doing high school physics class experiments amidst all the other classes that he didn't like left a lasting mark on Henry's preferred choice of learning list.

Such students "feel" their way through their activities, relying on an inner sense of what works for them. When allowed to follow this inner guidance system as adults, many an invention, creation, and original work have been the result. And how many of these people were ADD? Many!

As an addendum to this conclusion is the tendency of a high percentage of ADD people to not be drawn to "book learning." I'm not talking about whether a person is an avid reader or not; it appears that some are strong readers and others not so. But, the propensity to jump in and work directly with an idea is ADD. This often ties in with another ADD primary attribute, "Seeing the Big Picture" (chapter 1, table 1.1).

Henry and Patterns, Interconnections, and the Big Picture

Speaking of reading leads to the next early sign of ADD demonstrated by Henry when in early elementary school. At the time, he was trying to learn to read but not doing well considering his intelligence. As it turned out, he didn't have a diagnosable learning difference. Rather he needed to be given the tools to decipher the words that were hard for him to get his fingers around in order to understand them. (Interestingly, I initially wrote the word "fingers" to describe how he learned to understand how to read. Technically, fingers is the wrong word. Yet in retrospect, it was a very ADD way of describing the feeling of what happened for him, so I've decided to leave it as yet one more example of the style of ADD experiencing.)

He recalls how slow his learning to read was in contrast to how fast his kinesthetic learning allowed him to understand things en masse, as he gained understanding of the whole picture of much of what he was being taught. One of the first things the teacher did was break the teaching techniques into small bits that allowed him to see the parts of what he was trying to string together in order to get a Big Picture that made sense to him.

Partly, this problem with structuring the language in a way that he could understand was a precursor for his difficulties in structuring his creative, entrepreneurial, adult work projects. Once he saw not the words per se, but the patterns of the word combinations, he was able to read with increased efficiency. The biggest problem faced by Henry as he moved into adulthood stemmed from his ability to clearly see the Big Picture. In fact, he saw it so clearly, as in a dream at times, that he forgot that big pictures are made up of many small parts.

Granted, an Analogue person tends to see that Big Picture thanks to vision and creativity. But in order to implement the Big Picture, it is essential that the Big Picture be converted into a picture made up of its many parts. The whole picture will be in danger of falling apart if one tries to deal with it in one piece. Rather it probably needs to be disassembled and moved piece by piece.

Also of great importance is the ability to bring a creative vision into the everyday world of tangible, salable, replicable objects or processes to be sought by those wishing to buy it. There are details galore that must be lined up from production to marketing and sales, distribution, tracking, human resource management to . . . and so on. The initial visionary will have few of the skills needed after the first creative idea is acknowledged. That's when the whole thing can begin to break down.

In summary, the very skill that has been Henry's hallmark is also the very attribute that disallowed success because of his untrained ADD attributes. This is the key to learning to accommodate ADD that you'll read about in chapter 6.

Henry and His Strong Sensing Capability

Like many of us with an Analogue brainstyle, Henry had a strong sensate capability that operated, unknown to anyone around him, when he was young. Here's how it works: We tend to think first through our ability to *sense* what is going on both around us and within us rather than by thinking *about* what is happening.

His ADD sensing was well tuned even in childhood, becoming more so as the years went by. Though it took him a long time to trust what he felt, too often overriding his feelings for something that he thought he wanted or should do, he eventually began to learn self-trust so that he could get better control of his life. His sensing body is smarter than his thinking mind, which is true for many of us.

A High Level of Sensitivity

Always one to pick up on emotions as if he were a sponge, others' emotions had an immediate effect on Henry and the situations he faced day to day. When his tutor encouraged him, he wanted to try. He felt he had a colleague. He felt supported and guided, two factors that were key to his ADD nature.

Somehow, as adults lose track of understanding that we all do the best we can at a given moment, they also lose the gentle supportive nature that woos learners forward. Without that kind guidance, Henry lost a major support that guided him to walk a straight, productive path. Because of the fact that he didn't have a strong innate ability to structure the world around him, it was important as he went into adulthood to maintain an external source of guidance. He didn't have this, as you will shortly see.

Eventually Henry will have to replace the kindly math teacher with his own strong, caring adult self who will take care of the little child within him who is recovering from his losses with the help of the adult he's becoming.

The Adult Years

Only later in adulthood, the truth of his brainstyle and the potential for losses showed itself with a vengeance. Thus continues the story of the before, middle, and aftermath of a journey through the difficult territory of Attention Deficit Hyperactivity Disorder and the wisdom and insight that can be derived from the understanding of what can be achieved when ADD is embraced.

With psychological armor surrounding him, Henry went for broke when he was twenty-three years old. With spotty college credits and trial-and-error work ventures trailing behind his decision to commit to his dream, he felt it was the time to take a small delivery business into the big time. And this he did, taking control as he built his way to becoming the entrepreneur he wanted to become.

In Henry's own words, here's the story of his budding dream and its demise: "My dreams of greatness overtook my rational thought of taking my time in building a calculated plan. Because I am such a talented sales person, negotiator, and leader, I was able to overcompensate for my lack of structure . . . for a time, that is.

"At twenty-three, I took control and built a staff of thirty around me. I had my arms in everything and slowly started to lose control. I began to resent vendors and employees as I started getting further and further behind.

"I was bringing in a ton of business but couldn't understand why I wasn't making any real money. This led to a few years of major stress.

"Then I broke up with my girlfriend and started downhill. I was always positive, but I started to allow my deviant side to take over doing things that were maladaptive to make myself feel better and give myself a boost.

"I became manipulative (which turned out to mean that he made trades to get what he wanted) to satisfy the needs I couldn't satisfy. This led to legal trouble. No one got hurt, no drugs, but now I am on probation. I didn't mean to hurt anyone in anyway. I was just drowning in my emotions and needed help.

"I shut out my family and friends. During this time, I became hyper-focused on my business and nothing else mattered. I worked and came home. That's it. I was very lonely. There was no one in place to catch me."

Not able to trust friends, family, or colleagues and coworkers, he isolated himself from potential help. His sensitivity to what he perceived as criticism did not allow him to accept help. Later, though, he acknowledged those trying to talk with him may have been making suggestions.

After Henry lost the contract that fed his business, he was arrested. From there he ended up losing everything. At that point he turned a corner becoming introspective.

"I was propelled to take stock, which led me to finding a therapist who discovered my style of brain construction. I sought help to understand what happened, to change how I was, and to develop coping abilities. Now, I'm on a great, 'be careful' track and starting to learn how to change. I'm on my way to Self-Control."

You can read more about Henry and his healing and recovery in chapter 6.

Achieving Self-Control is worth the time and energy. The alternative is to live with a value system that you've not thought through. For your value system to not be one you've structured after you become an adult is worse. If you do what you think you *should* do rather than what you *want* to do, you will tend to feel resentful and/or depressed. On the other hand, if you *don't* do what you think you should do, you will end up feeling guilty. That means pain. Either way, you lose when your value system resides outside yourself. You will have no way to get to your *True Self*.

Under pressure, you won't be able to be counted on to act in a self-controlled way. You are likely to be suggestible. You will tend to cling to a belief proposed by another person. Many accomplices take this path and pay dearly for it. Placing the power of choice outside of yourself, ultimately, is a losing proposition.

Had Henry only known, he could have avoided a lot of heartache. But, rarely do we understand in our youth what we need to know. Add to that our ADHD style and we tend to be prone to want to get going. Talk about a setup to cause trouble; it behooves us to consider another major cause of difficulty—bad habits. You must commit to dealing with bad habits or you'll be fooling yourself that you can find and live the life of the wonderful person you're intended to be.

So let's take a look at some of the serious difficulties you face—*and can conquer*—in chapter 3.

3

BEING HELPED AND HELPING OTHERS

FROM WOUNDING TO GETTING HELP

We've been talking a lot about wounding—how it happens, what it looks like, and how to deal with it on your journey to finding and implementing your *True You*. Removing and reducing these larger blocks that hinder your being able to believe in yourself is paramount, because without doing it, you may be caught in an endless cycle of feeling as if there is something wrong with you.

Or, less formidable, you will be working way too hard to accomplish everything. You'll not feel hopeful that you'll find a path that opens before you so you can seek and find who you are and then implement your personal plan(s) for living the life you deserve and that fits you.

There are more strategies, skills, and aids that you can use to prepare yourself for a life that fits you—one that will bring joy and success to you.

After reviewing the interviews I've shared with you in the first chapters, I began noticing triggers and chuckholes that could get in the way of your healing journey: situations, issues (an issue creates a momentary show-stopper, but is not as serious as wounding), and snags on the *True You* Road.

After identifying wounding, it's time to clean up the mess, clear out the nonfunctional debris, and heal. In retrospect, I realize that I began to look at this section a bit like spring cleaning. It needs to be done so that your ADD self can work well, but it can be a bit tough. It's not HARD WORK, but it is work. Let's take a quick look at what we're going to cover. You may be surprised at what you find out.

First, we'll take a look at self-help interventions. We need to be able to tell the difference between the stress-related emotional upheaval of being ADD in a Linear culture and mental health conditions that have no connections with ADD. We'll look at mood and anxiety disorders, substance abuse, and serious psychological impairments.

The next section, Response to Trauma, covers the steps available for gaining help to heal serious abuse and neglect that has been a part of your growing-up experience.

A third wounding that must be attended to is Chronic Stress Response. Chronic stress is due to the wounding that results from living in a Linear culture. Though not caused directly by having an ADD brainstyle, it is a secondary wounding that is caused by a culture that *fits* a Linear processing person, but not one with an ADD brainstyle. This wounding can be greatly helped, so that your pathway to your *True You* can be cleared for easy travel.

Three additional subjects are covered in this chapter so that you will become free to move forward toward the embracing of your ADD.

- Diagnosis and Follow-Through: We'll sort out the issues that can come up in the identification of ADD: wounding, response to the labeling, and plans for management of this diversity brainstyle—plans that will benefit you rather than further entrap or wound you.

- Dealing with Fear: This normal emotion, though experienced both by ADD and non-ADD people, is all the more wounding when it has to do with whether an individual is deemed lesser than his peers or inadequate in some manner. A frequent participant in wounding responses of ADD, you will learn to curb the impact and free yourself of a major source of damage.

- Clearing Guilt: Forgiving yourself and changing values gives you a process to complete your growth, using the Core Components of Human Nature that we just discussed in chapter 2, so you can become Self-Controlled and guilt-free.

Self-Help

For nearly twenty years, my colleague Dr. John Rubel (the prison psychologist I introduced you to in chapter 1) and I have discussed common interests about ADD. As this book evolved in my mind, I would often discuss ideas with him. His input is always refreshing and insightful. Since he is a currently practicing mental health clinician with a strong ADD-as-a-Diversity bent, it was natural to talk with him about the Self Help section of this chapter. To that end, I want to share a particular conversation he and I had.

Lynn Weiss (LW): John, let's begin by talking about self-help as a way to work with ADD. What do you think about utilizing this mode of intervention?

John Rubel (JR): Self-help skill-building training and teaching are actually a preferred intervention for mentally healthy people with an Analogue brainstyle. Training programs have been used for a long time. New variations are in the making in which those who are more experienced with management of their own ADD will work with and support others through teaching and coaching accommodation skills.

Cognitive-emotional-behavioral skills can be passed along the chain, with peers driving accommodation. Thus you're working with like-kind mentors who intuit or know from experience what you may need to escape from the murky waters of the Linear world. There's not an "I know the answer" attitude. Instead, both companionship and the sharing of accommodations are more likely to be a good fit for your brainstyle. As a result, you are more likely to avoid accumulation of chronic stress.

By creating and maintaining a strong, encouraging social support network, you receive an additional circle of protection for you and your ADD-way. Thus you become a part of the ADD perspective to the degree to which it is beneficial to you as like-kind help like-kind.

LW: John, I'd like your take on the relationship between ADD and general clinical psychological issues.

JR: Brainstyle is only one of many aspects that make up each of us. We need to explain to newcomers to the world of ADD—as well as anyone else you get hold of—that "ADD is a diversity issue, not a pathological condition."

Whether we are ADD (Analogue) or non-ADD (Linear), we may have blue eyes or brown, pale skin or dark, a "type A" high strung personality or a "type B" easy-going personality. None of this is abnormal or pathological. So, it's likely that you won't need to do much about the way you're made, other than adjusting to *fit* environments that don't readily enhance your natural way of being.

LW: So where do things go so terribly wrong for so many people with an ADD brainstyle?

JR: Regardless of one's brainstyle, life is full of problems and stress, especially if a person lives in an invalidating environment. If you have an ADD brainstyle, over time you may develop situational symptoms from the wounding that occurs from your environment. Let's say that on the job you are expected to learn and work in a Linear, abstract manner sitting down at a desk. But as a part of your ADD attributes, you learn kinesthetically (hands-on) by actively manipulating your "tools," be they numbers or words. You may use tangible demonstration, storytelling, or modeling to do the job, rather than sitting at a table reading about or tallying numbers in columns.

Because the *fit* is often poor between your learning methodology and the one that is required, you likely have become stressed. As stress builds, you may develop a cluster of symptoms that qualifies for a psychiatric diagnosis such as mood disorders, anxiety disorder, substance abuse disorder, or some other serious problem that impacts your ability to function across a variety of situations.

LW: Depression is a prevalent condition that affects many people. And many people with an ADD brainstyle have had to deal with depression. How do you see the connection?

JR: No one would argue that severe clinical depression is a serious mind-body illness. But is having an ADD brainstyle a serious mind-body illness? Remember if you have an ADD brainstyle and find yourself in a situation that is a good *fit* for your brainstyle, you excel; if you find yourself in a situation that is a bad *fit*, you struggle. Your performance varies based on your environment's goodness of *fit*.

LW: Many people with an ADD brainstyle are told, "If you only do it this way you would be more successful." I've noticed that frequently the individual has tried and tried to do it in the way suggested. What have you noticed in these situations?

JR: First and foremost, depression, often existing at a moderate level, is often jolted by the latest attempt to help an ADD person. Frequently framed as a "suggestion," they are often heard as a last chance for hope in an impossible situation. Being asked to try something that has resulted in failure more times than anyone can count only floods the person's emotional system even further. Feelings of failure and hopelessness—key components of depression—move in to increase the depth of the feelings.

What works for a person with a non-ADD brainstyle doesn't work for a person with an ADD brainstyle. And what works for one ADD brainstyle might not work for another. What works for one type of ADD may not work for another type. But most people don't know this—even clinically and educationally trained people don't seem to know it.

You and I know that the type of training that works for an Olympic sprinter won't work for a marathon runner. Although there may be some similarities in their training routines, the majority of their training is very different. It's as simple as that.

LW: What about conditions such as anxiety, behavioral problems, addiction, and serious mental health conditions?

JR: I would be remiss if I didn't tell you that just because you're ADD doesn't mean that you also may not have an emotionally based condition, mental illness, or personality disorder that needs attention. Signs that may raise physical and mental concerns include severe depression, anxiety, chronic emotional and interpersonal problems, substance abuse and impulse control problems.

LW: What special guidelines would you suggest about dealing with ADD and addictions?

JR: When chemical dependency and other addiction issues are involved, you must, unequivocally, be in treatment for them and abstaining from behavior that is problematic. It is helpful to simultaneously take your brainstyle into account. But your addiction must *always* be front and center in your treatment program. ADD is no excuse for addictive disorders to continue or for you to fail to actively treat any active addiction in which you are involved. None!

LW: What should someone with an ADD brainstyle expect when seeking mental health counseling?

JR: It's important to find a mental health professional who can attend to your mental health needs without causing further wounding to you due to a lack of understanding that ADD is a diversity issue, not a medical or pathological disorder that needs to be corrected. The counselor needs to have training and/or experience with someone who knows the boundaries between mental health and diversity.

The majority of medically trained practitioners have been taught that ADD is a mental health disorder; something is wrong with you that requires fixing. Even when the mental health professional is empathetic, you may be exposed to an implicit message that the professional knows better than you.

LW: What else can help find the right person to counsel you?

JR: One way to protect your Wounded You is to have a frank and open discussion about how you see your ADD brainstyle. Notice the reaction of the listener while you listen to that intuitive voice inside your mind that lets you know if this person is safe for you to work with. If you do not feel comfortable and validated by a mental health professional, continue your search until you find one that is a good fit for you.

Psychotherapy is an effective and powerful treatment when you need more than teaching and training to both effectively use your ADD style in a Linear world and protect against wounding from a lack of *fit*.

LW: What about being a self-advocate in relation to ADD?

JR: The world of Attention Deficit Disorder in adults is complex and is just now being seen and understood to be the diversity issue that it is. By following the field research of those with this Analogue style of brain construction, guidelines are emerging that are teaching the truth about what ADD is and what it isn't.

Individuals with ADD attributes are on the front line of understanding. Each in his or her own way are passing on a new perspective that allows people of any brainstyle to be valuable and needed to balance our culture.

Through teaching, training, and mentoring of this new perspective, the pathologizing and medicalizing of this created disorder is changing. In dealing with a major mind-body illness we are all learning to work together. Self-help and learning from those farther down the road than ourselves joins teachers, mentors, and coaches to make headway in the managing of ADD in the twenty-first century.

In addition, we can now partner with medical professionals to distinguish mind-body illness from Chronic Stress Response due to ADD wounding. We can improve in both separating ADD from the medical model, while simultaneously dealing with major mental health issues.

Together, we are on our way to striving to be who we were always meant to be: our *True Selves*.

Response to Trauma (PTSD)

Being ADD is not a traumatic event. You can have an ADD brainstyle, however, and also have a traumatic event. They begin as two separate events or situations each different from the other. You can have one or many traumas from childhood, as shown in Alphonso's story.

Alphonso was the only son of an alcoholic father and immigrant mother. His mother stayed home until his sister reached school age and then began to do housework to make enough money to make up for the amount that her husband drank weekly. Al was nine at the time.

Al was an active boy, smart enough, but not a very good student. His mother wasn't able to help him, though she wished she could, but her schooling had been short lived. His little sister scooted quietly around the house so as not to draw attention to herself. But Alphonso, no matter how hard he tried, always seemed to be bumping into things, spilling drinks on the floor, and generally acting like a boy.

He learned early that he should stay out of the way of his father—who was already drunk when he arrived home after work
and didn't stop drinking all evening. The more he drank, the
meaner he got. He blamed everything that he thought was wrong
with his life on his family: his job, having to share the money he
made with his family, a kid who reminded him of how he was
raised in poverty and abuse, and a wife whom he thought was
inferior to him, reflecting his inability to attract someone of value.

Al, his mom, and sister would spend the evening in the kids'
bedroom to stay out of the way of the old man. When Al got home
from after-school activities, his mom would try to shield him from
his father so that he'd be safe—safe from becoming a battering
post for his father's rage and pain. Al felt his father's anger until his
mom managed to grab him away while her husband was pouring
yet another drink.

This was the story that Alphonso, now a man in his thirties, told
me after I'd talked with him several times. He had begun drinking
to try to block out his own emotional pain and fear that he had carried into adulthood. Now he was in an alcohol recovery program
that was meant to help him stop drinking and reduce his fear. He
met Henry (chapter 2, p. 71) who already was working with his
own issues of ADD, and recognized that Al had many of the same
attributes that he had. He thought Al might benefit from learning
more about his brainstyle.

I had noticed in the first three visits that Al was not very trusting of the idea that he could find help for himself. He barely
spoke. He was self-effacing and was not comfortable with the
reading and writing that he was facing in his treatment group,
which at the time was a group exercise in a rehab class he was
taking. He didn't think much of himself. He had little self-worth.

Yet I noticed that behind the resistance to suggestions of what
he could do to handle his ADD, a small glimmer of understanding began to emerge. In fact, he demonstrated intelligence that

wasn't well educated, but seemed innate. He always seemed to understand what I was saying.

Finally, on the fourth visit, he suddenly said, "I think I was an okay kid until the day that my dad came home a little early." Then Al told me his story. "I was ten, and my mom wasn't home yet. Before I knew what happened, my dad strong-armed me into his room and locked the door from the inside. He began to hit me, beat me, and yell at me. I couldn't understand him and didn't know what he was talking about. He'd whipped me lots of times before and even beat on me—but always before, my mother would rush in to save me even if it meant that she got hit, which happened a lot. But this time, she couldn't get in when she returned home. My dad had locked the door of his room. Nothing could save me.

"I don't know how long he raged and yelled and hit and spat on me. And I don't know why, but I know that I didn't wake up for hours and couldn't go to school the next day. All I know is that I still have nightmares about the beating by him. I can smell the alcohol and sweat even now when I'm alone at night. I never went near him again.

"I'm afraid to try to do anything because I won't be able to get it right. I'm no more able to do anything right now that I'm grown than I could then."

Alphonso lived with the memories of the giant trauma that had been surrounded by smaller traumas and fears of traumas repeating themselves through his life—in truth and in his inner world of memories.

Attention Deficit Disorder didn't create Alphonso's traumatic childhood. Nor did his traumatic beatings and home environment create his ADD. But they were long ago woven together into a tangled web that it's now time to unweave, as he judiciously is willing to trust just a little bit to see what he can do with the rest of his life.

Let's begin by building an understanding of what happened to Alphonso. Then we can reverse the process and rebuild again in a healthy way.

Remember how Trust is the first Core Component of Human Nature that a child must build in order to feel that he will get his needs met? In this case, it was a need for safety and security. In a violent or traumatic situation—whether it happens just once or more than once—safety and security are jeopardized and remain impaired during subsequent years until intervention helps us deal with the loss of trust that we'll be safe from harm. Consider the following Response to Trauma (nature, war, family, severe loss, and hurts of all kinds):

- The Event creating the Trauma happens.
- Immediately—whether the trauma is a beating or a rape, a hurricane that destroys our home or the violent death of a loved one—Safety is Lost.
- A Grief Reaction automatically occurs, sliding into our emotional environment.
- We go through The Five Stages of Grief (which generally occur repeatedly and may or may not happen in an orderly manner)

    ○ Disbelief
    ○ Anger
    ○ Guilt
    ○ Depression
    ○ Acceptance

The last stage is the time when healing (which usually takes at least a minimum of two years) reaches acceptance of the loss. This does not mean that the loss is forgotten. Rather, the loss is accepted so that life can continue to grow. Slowly, new beginnings, laughter, and hope return with a renewal for the self. The individual is, of course, a changed person who has had a traumatic loss or event. But after acceptance, you will also be able to grow again as you once did prior to the loss.

At the time of the trauma, a Regression Response usually happens. Emotionally, victims regress to a younger stage of development. For example, if you had a moderate level of Self Control, you would likely feel inadequate as if you no longer had control or powerfulness or even competence. You might feel as if your whole world might splinter, leaving even your identity shattered. And you might find it hard to trust anyone until you were helped to heal.

In the case of severe trauma, violence, pain, and fear, the hurt can continue for years, often evolving into Post Traumatic Stress Disorder (PTSD).

In cases of traumatic loss, symptoms soon seem to bring the experience of Hitting Bottom. In that state, feelings of helplessness and/or hopelessness usually occur so that loss of a Sense of Trust and Identity trigger depression, anger, and fear of never being normal again.

In this state, we tumble down, down, down to the bottom of the barrel before we can begin to recover and move back toward health. It's likely to be a long way up, but one of the most important supports is to have someone aware of the challenges you face and what they mean because that person has been there personally. Each of us needs the educated support of another person who walks their talk.

No matter what our age—whether we are a child, teen, young adult, middle adult, or elder—we still need what we need when we need it in order to recover. Usually that means help. The order in which we receive the help is important.

First, we need Protection (child or adult): Someone to be with us on our journey and to provide safety.

Second, we need an Expression of Grief: Someone who conveys compassion and says, "I'm sorry, you didn't deserve what happened to you."

Now we can begin to rebuild our feelings of competence—at first with the help of another and eventually on our own.

Our job becomes the Rebuilding of the Core Components of Human Nature, one at a time. Do not be in any rush. Everyone has his or her own timing. On your own, you will:

First: Rebuild Trust.

Second: Gently allow Separation from the person who's been helping you.

Third: You will refashion your Identity; you are now someone who has had the trauma as a part of your life.

Fourth: Reinforce your Sense of Competence. You can take little steps. You can manage small gains, even as small as getting out of bed in the beginning. Increasingly, you will be able to take bigger steps and become competent again.

Fifth: Give yourself permission to be Powerful. Your caregiver must give you back your power so that your healing becomes your own.

Sixth: You will rejoice in your Self-Control once again. Celebrate your achievements.

Days, weeks, months or even years—it doesn't matter how long it takes to recover. Encourage this cycle to be completed, but don't rush it. Even after years, you may have flashbacks and dreams that remind you of the terrible thing that happened that one time, or those several or many times. But either way, you can brave the storm with help from others who have been there before you.

The reason this is important for you as someone with ADD is that one of the main attributes of ADD is Sensitivity. Unfortunately, this attribute lays us wide open to be directly hurt or to absorb the pain from others' traumas. Even group traumas, such as natural disasters and television news coverage, can expose ADD people to undue stress. We don't automatically compartmentalize our hurt and pain, which in the long run makes us more vulnerable than many of our friends and family, but also gives us the opportunity to ultimately help and heal others.

With extra "padded" support and care during the healing phase, we can become truly compassionate people who become great helpers, healers, and protectors, passing on our own experiences. We may never forget what happened, but we *can* reclaim our lives.

Chronic Stress Response (CSR)

As you've seen, wounding comes in many forms. Sometimes it is a one-shot big wound from a hurt, loss, or disappointment. That's usually called a "traumatic event" and can leave the victim with PTSD: Post Traumatic Stress Disorder. But there's another kind of wounding that has a different kind of design.

It's a slow-building, incessant series of let-downs, "not quites," and self-critical disappointments from dreaming more than could be accomplished. Chronic Stress Response (CSR) comes from being blamed for things you have had no control over. It may be the result of trying as hard as you could and still failing to reach a goal that you wanted. It's finding yourself jealous of what others are able to achieve when you feel that you're at least as smart as they are.

It feels like you are not only letting everyone else down but, worse yet, you are letting yourself down. And you ask that self, "How is it possible to dream something that I can't make happen?" You know you're not dumb, but you don't achieve, nor are you recognized for the incredible originality and visions you have in your mind.

You may notice that you don't get over a feeling of being "less than." Your self-worth may be in the cellar, except every once in a while when you have a new idea or opportunity. At that moment, you may feel that, "This time will be different." This time, you feel so wonderfully right about what you want that you are certain that you'll be able to pull it off.

But, when you don't pull it off and the same old sadness begins to creep back in as you realize you're not going to be able to reach the goals that you feel but can't touch, you begin to get that gut-wrenching sense in the pit of your stomach and tears well up in your eyes. Depression isn't far behind. And there you are, sliding down on the slippery slope to hopelessness.

Or if your personality is more outgoing, you may take a different route. First you announce your new dream idea to the whole world, shouting it from the mountain top. Then as others don't cluster around you to congratulate you on your brilliance and high level of creativity, you begin to feel shame. The more you realize what isn't happening, the more you become angry at those who are ignoring you—as if it is their fault. You may blame anyone who you dreamed might be able to help you and hasn't come forward.

You likely become a rumbling volcano that isn't far from exploding at any given time as you bury your feelings of sadness and hopelessness, making enough noise to scare away the outcome that you don't want. Alcohol or another excess may become your best friend at this time.

The repeated hopefulness of the dream to which we reach, followed by the dreadful failure to achieve it for reasons we don't understand is a setup for joyful, passionate emotions at the beginning of a project or goal to turn into desperate, wretched grief when we cannot ignore our failure. The result creates a mood swing that has often been diagnosed as manic depression. Unlike the biochemical bipolar disorder, however, this mood swing is situational—dependent upon the way we humans react to hope and failure.

One of my personal most memorable, repeating cycles happened every time I started a new class in school. I'd get the book(s) before the class started, I'd excitedly sit down to read in order to get ahead, even when I was a young student. I'd research the subject matter and the next thing I knew, the semester was partially over and I was way behind in the reading, and busy creating ways to finish assignments in whatever way I could. (Mostly I creatively made projects, spent a lot of time with the teachers talking about the subject, and worked far more hours than any school kid ought to.)

Then I didn't know why I got the results I did, even if I received an A, because I couldn't master the topic in a Linear way that looked smart. So I felt more and more horrible and depressed as the semester unfolded, after having been very excited about learning new things in the beginning. I loved learning new things; I just didn't like the process of learning them.

For years after my schooling was over, I had nightmares about getting behind in college and it was time for the finals—except then I'd awaken feeling sick and realize I'd already graduated from college and didn't even need the courses. How sad! Only in writing this book did I finally realize what the repetitive dream was about. Whew, I'm glad it's done for.

These scenarios repeated over time create Chronic Stress Response because of the many times that the pattern of eager hope and frustrated disappointment has occurred—starting in the early school years and continuing through your later education and into adulthood, as you face the work world that continues to cause similar troubles.

Many times you and I and all our kindred spirits have been the victim of not *fitting* into the way in which goals are reached in this culture. As someone with ADD struggling to reach your potential in a significantly Linear culture, you have faced a mammoth task that requires understanding the reason(s) why you struggle to succeed.

It is the accumulation of little and moderate-sized frustrations experienced over and over that has set you up to begin to react when you feel the very first reminder of the sequence that has been repeated so many times. Without meaning to, you've memorized the top of the slippery slope so much that feeling it instantly brings the whole ride down to mind, along with the terrible feelings that are waiting at the bottom. Chronic Stress Response has arrived at your doorstep.

It can be at this point that the response to the hurt and loss brings you in contact with the medical profession. Those who practice within the medical model tend to contrast health with a disease or deficiency disorder, such as: oppositional defiant behavior, emotional intensity disorder, impulse regulation disorder, or emotional dis-regulation disorder. Depression and anger disorders also are usually diagnosed at this time for, to be sure, that is what you are demonstrating. And they are linked to your brainstyle name with the term "comorbidity." This labels both your brainstyle and the resultant repetitive wounding as diseased and/or disordered when, in actuality, neither is the case.

I recall one conference in the mid-1990s when I questioned the speaker at the podium in an attempt to create a dialogue about the relationship between ADD and depression. The point I wanted to make was, "How can you have an ADD style of brain construction in this culture and not be depressed or enraged?" Their relationship is a matter of cause and effect, not comorbidity. The discussion did not occur at that time. But, perhaps there will be another chance, thanks to you and me. Sometimes we have to wait a long time to get our just due.

As I've sought to find a label to deal with the issues of deep wounding reactions, I spoke again with my colleague, Dr. John Rubel. "I think," he said, "What you're describing and searching to find a label for is the result of an individual, regardless of brainstyle, whose mind/body has been in chronic stress. Whatever a person's genetic vulnerabilities are, being in a chronic stress response will ultimately turn on those genes and over time, symptoms develop that eventually lead to a healthcare professional giving a diagnosis, a label, to a mind/body illness.

"ADD brainstyle individuals are more likely to experience a CSR in modernized Western industrial societies because of the increased frequency of invalidating environments to which they are exposed. This will continue until our society appreciates and values brainstyle diversity."

Let me tell you, this instantly explained the essence of a deep internal sense of "wrongness" that pervades our self-esteem, blurs our belief in ourselves, and drains our energies—including the hopes and dreams and physical fortitude to follow what is our passion.

What we need to do is challenge the belief that we are some-how abnormal and replace it with the belief that we are absolutely right for who we are. There isn't, never was, and never will be anything *wrong* with us simply because we have an ADD style of brain construction. Until I discovered ADD in my own self, I had felt that something was *wrong* with me at the deepest level of my being. It was my secret for over fifty years.

We must, however, approach our learning and our work in ways that *fit* us, and find the accommodations that *fit* us in accomplishing the tasks of our choice, free of a predominantly Linear learning and accomplishment style to the exclusion of Analogue learning and evaluation techniques. Evaluations of our abilities must be achieved through demonstration and other Analogue methods rather than Linear goal-testing to prove that we know what we know or can do what we can do.

And we must demand this not only from the society at large, but from ourselves—we who have succumbed to the values and beliefs of the predominantly Linear culture that has the institutional power to say who does what and how—in order for the doors of learning and success to open.

A little or a lot of self-brainwashing is necessary to turn this situation around. Each of us can do it for ourselves and we can help one another. Perhaps we need a motto such as the one African Americans conjured to change their self-perception: "Black is Beautiful." Anyone have a slogan?

"DIAGNOSIS" VERSUS "IDENTIFICATION:" FOLLOW-THROUGH AND AFTERCARE

A little over a year ago, I received an email from Mari H. She'd found my book, *Attention Deficit Disorder in Adults* (4th edition) at her local library. She wrote, after being evaluated for ADD, "I wish I'd found your book years ago. I am living a miserable life. But I now understand the labels, 'overactive,' 'sensitive,' 'very imaginative,' etc. They used to mean something different than they do now. It was like something was *wrong* with me."

I responded to her by affirming how hard it is to be misunderstood, but that lots of us recover and become happy being who we really are, naturally. Her next sentence made my heart feel sad.

"At fifty-five, there's probably not too much that can be done for me, but I will see if there are any organizations locally that may be able to assist me to accept who and what I am and help me feel better."

"So young!" I thought. I affirmed her seeking support and needing mentors and models to follow, at least for a while. I suggested a couple more books and reminded her once more that she is valuable. And I encouraged her to stay in touch.

I did not hear from Mari for nearly a year. But, since I make a habit of responding to meaningful dialogues, I checked in with her for an update. Two days later I received her reply.

"I must admit, my ADD 'slapped me right in the face' last year." Then she added, "Amazingly enough, the information I have gleaned from reading your books helped prevent a major depressive episode."

Oh my, I thought. How glad I am that she was able to stem the tide of her hurt, frightened feelings by connecting a lifeline to the words I'd written. From this, we began to dialogue throughout my writing of this book, with more of her story unfolding over time.

It seems that her reaction to being assessed for ADD revealed an inherent flaw in the process that too often surfaces, setting her fear response in action. In her situation, she was "diagnosed" by her general practitioner and left with no follow-up. So, it was verified that there was "something wrong with her," which she already believed. But there was no further information or planning to show her the way out. She saw herself as a "lifer," someone living the rest of her life with no hope for parole.

Too often, the aftermath of an ADD assessment or testing leaves an individual with little or no follow-up. It doesn't seem to matter whether the evaluation comes from a professional, a medical doctor, a psychologist, a psychiatrist, a licensed counselor, an educator, or a magazine checklist.

Another post-assessment scenario that isn't helpful is the prescription of medication for ADD with no behavioral guidance or accommodation training or education about what it means in the broad picture to be made with the brainstyle diversity called ADD. People working in the field of ADD have known for years that medication without education and training has no better results, or is even worse, than doing nothing to assist a person in dealing with their brainstyle.

Many people whom I've seen over the years have self-diagnosed. Observing or recognizing your brainstyle naturally leads to reaching out for information, which is what you need. That's what Mari did.

My experience is that formal "therapy" is rarely the answer. Why? Because ADD is not a "something's wrong with me that needs to be fixed" issue. What *is* needed is a heightened awareness of what ADD really is, how it works, its assets and liabilities in particular situations, how to find situations that *fit*, or how to accommodate it when you're faced with a misfitting environment in which you choose to remain.

You and Mari and all of us need to learn about how we're made with all our assets and liabilities.

You will want to find your specialness that is due to your particular style of brain construction. You need not pay a lot of money to accomplish this. By being discriminating as you read, using the aspects of the educational system that understand kinesthetic learning, and making use of trial-and-error observation, you'll be able to be who you were always meant to be.

As Dr. Rubel so clearly points out, you must sort out "other" issues from ADD. Standalone ADD doesn't need therapy, but ADD can surely be negatively affected in the context of "other" issues.

What's afterwards—after the discovery of ADD and the sorting out of Dr. Rubel's points—turns out to be extremely important. It will determine how you see yourself and whether you rise above a belief about yourself that no longer diminishes you. Mari seems to be sufficiently free of other issues to move forward. In chapter 6, p. 188, you will discover how she learned to make the appropriate accommodations.

As I've watched the many scenarios that have unfolded the last thirty-plus years, I've come to the conclusion that informal education and training and personal observations top the list for successful transitioning to being who you can be with your ADD-ways and skills.

You must observe what you like and don't like, what you do easily and find difficult, and most of all what is pleasurable as you discover and allow yourself to live out the dreams of your lifetime. Then you focus on learning to accommodate your brainstyle for use in Linear situations that you've decided are a part of your *True Self*. Finally, you can then decide if medication would help you in the short term or long term as you work with your accommodation training.

Mari's next email told me that she had the self-observation skills necessary to find her path. Her email told me also that she was a perfect candidate to use the Dialogue Approach of Mentoring that would lead her to desired results that *fit* her, even from a long distance.

The Email Dialogue Approach in an
ADD Mentoring Program

The update that yielded a better history of Mari's current situation served to jump-start a whole new approach to working with mentally healthy people who happen to have an ADD style of brain construction. Neither Mari nor any of us is perfect, and I promise you we all have our "issues." But the depression that dogged her prior to beginning her work with ADD was simply a situational depression—the result of the frustration from Chronic Stress Response and loss of hope that things would ever get better. It was the depression that is a part of the grief cycle that accompanies losses.

In this case, she was weighed down by the loss of hope that somehow she would ever be able to feel good about herself and the grief of being criticized and working below her insight and intelligence levels—losses that had weighed her down for fifty-five years and seemed intolerable if no hope was in sight. It was then that the door opened as we continued our online dialogue about her ADD.

In the same email in which Mari talked about feeling "slapped in the face with ADD," she continued, saying, "It's so nice to hear from you. I am currently enrolled in a business college. I realized I was never going to be successful working at a job I was not suited for. I am taking a Microsoft Office Certification course as well as QuickBooks. Looking back, I was always very successful working in a busy office environment, and a dismal failure in the telephone customer service arena. I felt like a 'caged animal' sitting in that tiny cubicle, tethered to a telephone with no human contact. Providing the same 'scripted' answers day after day was utterly miserable for me. I actually 'enjoy' having to 'think on my feet' from time to time!

"Hopefully I will be able to obtain suitable employment when I finish my course. [And she has.] Your books have helped me greatly. I was able to determine my strengths and weaknesses, and determine what environments are completely wrong for me.

"I hope you are well and I look forward to reading your new book. I understand now that ADD is not a disease."

I heard from Mari again within a few weeks via social media. My response to her was sent via email as I preferred at the time not to use social media. I wrote: "Mari, I am most happy to stay in touch with you. But at the moment, I'm not using any of the social media because checking it takes too much of my time when I'm in this period of intense focusing on writing. I'm also not drawn to it. However, any time you want to connect by email, I'd be happy to respond, Lynn."

Within a short time, I received the following email from Mari. I awaited it with interest, because Mari's response would let me check yet another time regarding the health of our email dialogue. She said, "This makes me feel better! The business school I am attending encourages students to have an 'Internet presence,' but I find it much too overwhelming. My mind is already trying to do a dozen things at once. I haven't been on social media for several years. I still prefer regular email or the telephone."

So there she was—discovering that someone else had similar feelings and responses to hers. That's what mentorship is. I knew then that we were operating on a horizontal plane and that it was valid, person-to-person, because Mari wasn't disordered or in need of my "protection." She didn't need to be dependent upon me. Therefore, a dialogue was appropriate.

My response ratcheted the dialogue up another notch: "You know, Mari, I struggled long and hard, all the time feeling guilty as well as feeling put down by others in my field, about exactly the way you are feeling. Going against general information from educators, professionals, and the public is difficult. Finally, I just decided I had to do things the way that was comfortable for me. I was neither interested in creating chaos and confusion nor feeling depressed and anxious because I wasn't ready to figure out how to use social media.

"I really admire you for being honest to my note and taking it as it was meant, having nothing to do with whether I was willing to communicate with you or not. [This was a major sign of her healthy thinking.] And thank you for being willing to join the system that I need in order to continue this dialogue with you."

Thus, the Dialogue Approach to Mentoring was affirmed, thanks to the interviews by email, phone, and in person.

I had already conceptualized a style of working that would follow up the identification of ADD brainstyles—an organic, natural program style that would provide resources to heal, grow, and excel in our own right. Not a rehab program, or a correctional program, but one that would pass accommodations, skills, and support—mentor to mentor—as we each learn from those who have gone before us. Then we pass on to those who follow, at the same time that we learn with, and from, them.

For the time being I am going to leave Mari, but you'll have two more chances to watch her progress before the end of this book. I'm happy to say that she is a mentor in the making.

OVERCOMING FEAR

Fear is not a comfortable feeling. But it is an ongoing part of life. It has a good side and a bad side. So we might as well get used to it, and figure out some things we can do about managing fear so it works in our best interest. Then we must learn to release it when it is playing the role of a "Trickster" with memories from our past or when getting us to listen to a system—like an educational system or culture or another person—telling us something that really isn't true for us.

The Trickster is a character in Native American mythology that works to teach by showing that we may be doing the exact opposite of what is best for us. Why? Because we're ceding our power to someone else's belief or instructions when it doesn't *fit* us or isn't in our best interest. Or maybe we are doing the very opposite of something that would be right for us.

Perhaps we learned we are not very smart because we never made it to the gifted and talented programs in our school. But what we didn't realize was that our diverse ADD brainstyle wasn't being accommodated in a strictly rigid Linear system. The way we were being taught didn't *fit* us. We simply needed to be taught in a different way. In reality, we were and are smart. But instead, we believed in what others thought and became afraid we weren't smart and wouldn't be able to become successful in life, become popular, or be able to do what we really want to do.

The second part of Trickster energy is to learn the value of laughter. Being too serious is believed to unbalance a person. Both seriousness and laughter are healthier, making one balanced. Opposites and humor are teaching tools and living skills.

Fear can play this role in our lives when we believe something is dangerous when, in reality, it is not. It may instead be a belief that someone else believes in but it is not fitting for us.

To be sure, there are times when we need to be afraid—such as when an eighteen-wheeler is careening out of control toward you. Please *do* let the fear propel you out of the way!

But often we are afraid because we are trying to do something that isn't good for us. It serves the purpose of warning us that our situation is either dangerous, or no good for us. Perhaps the timing of what we're trying to do is off. Maybe in a new business or project we get a strange feeling that makes us uncomfortable. You better begin to look for what's off about the situation. Unless you're a chronic, seriously frightened person, you can bet that something is amiss with an aspect of the business development: personnel, finances, timing, or hidden agendas behind the scenes.

Another scenario built upon a base of fear comes from memories registered in our youngest years. It certainly happened to me. I was raised by a mother who lived throughout her life with fears of all kinds. Her own background included being the oldest daughter of poor immigrant parents. Of eleven children, only four were known to grow to adulthood. One more appeared sixty-five years later, having suffered amnesia and been presumed dead for forty years.

It was hard not to be afraid when the family sometimes had to dig potatoes at a neighboring farm after dark so there would be something to eat that night. It's hard not to be afraid when you're very bright, extremely sensitive, and pulled out of school in the fifth grade to go to work for twenty-five cents a day, taking care of another family's children even after the local teacher begged your parents to let you remain in school. Add to that multiple personal hurts and injuries beyond your control, and you end up as a person whose world perspective is of a glass half empty, not half full.

The depth of my mother's level of deprivation and helplessness led to "learned fear"—fear of scarcity and fear of trying, hoping, or trusting that there was safety anywhere to be had. My mother's Sense of Trust was minute. Her Self-Esteem and Sense of Competence never developed, much less any ability to self-protect (Sense of Powerfulness). The latter tended to draw harmful situations to her. She had no grounds for judging people and was easily victimized, which only proved that the way she felt was indeed the way things were and would always be.

My mother—who had an ADD brainstyle although that was not known at the time—lived in a world of fantasy, for she had no sense of self that awaited her as the intelligent, attractive, and creative person she could have been. She had no chance to go further down the path to find her *True Self*, filled as she was with fear from the day she was born to the day she died eighty-nine years later.

In comparison, Mari's Sense of Trust that developed in her childhood allowed her to stay with her office training studies even when the going was hard. She felt nervous. But she kept going and did finish, and we'll hear more about that in chapter 6.

The point is this: It is so important when working with ADD, or any brainstyle, really, to be clear about the emotional underpinnings of the inner child when seeking to embrace one's ADD or get at the truth. Start with building your own or another's trust. Don't let yourself be pushed, and don't push someone you're mentoring.

One of the most effective tools in dealing with fear is demonstrating patience to calm a situation down. And one of the best ways to achieve patience is to use your breath and encourage others to use theirs. Assuming that the proverbial wild dog is not nipping at your heels, slow down. If you're working with someone else, demonstrate a slower breathing cycle. Also with yourself, take in a deep breath and then gently and smoothly release it totally. Repeat this controlled breathing and you'll begin to help yourself or another person get regrounded or stabilized.

Much of the fear that you suffer in situations where your ADD comes into play—as in classrooms, when projects need finishing, when you wonder if you will be able to do a good enough job because, after all, you never have been able to work up to your potential, never could manage time, etc., etc.—actually takes place in your head.

Let's do a little analysis. Think about the last time you felt fearful. What were you thinking about? Ah, thinking, right there in your head. Or remembering an earlier time when things didn't come off right. Fear pops up that you'll revisit that failure again. Okay, I said the dastardly word, "failure." Neither thinking about nor feeling fears of failure are "grounding."

Instead, fear underrides destabilization. And no one can think or feel emotionally stable if they feel unsafe. This is one of the most prevalent conditions that hounds most of us with an ADD style of brain.

What To Do About Destabilization and Fear and What Not To Do

I'll never forget hearing a community-based talk about fear in which the speaker asked for volunteers. A young lady, probably in her early twenties, volunteered. She was shy and uncomfortable about speaking in front of an audience. The leader believed that the way around this was to "force" her to face the feared situation. Rather than encouraging her with firm but kind support, he thought he needed to browbeat her, nearly yelling at her. She quickly acquiesced to stop the onslaught. It happened to be a time in our culture where force was a popular technique being used to break down people in the name of healing. I'd heard about it before seeing it used, didn't like it then, and didn't like it any better with the young woman as victim.

Not long after that I had occasion to be involved with addiction counseling and codependency. What I noticed was that there was a 180-degree difference in response to harsh rules between those in treatment for addiction and their spouses or family members.

I tended to agree that a very healthy setting of limits and insistence on abstinence was crucial to recovery for addicts. The recovering addicts tended to do well with extreme firmness and "loving" harshness. But I also noticed the effect of force and pressure on the spouses and nonchemically addicted family members. The latter did not do well in response to force and pressure.

The family members often did not have self-preservation techniques or a Sense of Powerfulness to self-protect in the first place, and they often lost gains they'd made previously. In the situations I'm talking about, they were victims, not perpetrators. And, too often, they came away from treatment programs broken down rather than stabilized and strengthened to set the necessary limits needed to regain *their* health, so they could move toward improvement in their relationship if that was to be possible.

As my work with ADD progressed and I saw the attribute of sensitivity that is so prevalent in many of us, I gained understanding of what works best to strengthen our true Sense of Powerfulness while learning to break free from playing out the addiction patterns.

When fear is present, remember to breathe. Remember to slow down. And gently increase the building of a true Sense of

Powerfulness as protection for your ADD sensitivity. Be firm with yourself. Be firm with others. Be consistent. Be self-protective and learn how to say, "No" and "That's enough for now."

As you gain emotional strength, there are several ways to begin to face fear head on. For example, let's say that you are worried about talking to your boss, a parent, or any authority.

First: Request a period of time to speak with the person. Specify the time limit and initially make it short.

Second: If you are sensitive to criticism, ask your boss to tell you what he or she does want and like rather than what wasn't liked. Then you can stretch to give what is wanted. That way you will feel confident instead of afraid of doing something *wrong*.

Third: Clarify what you want when you request an audience with your boss. Don't try to solve more than one issue at a time. If you have multiple issues, set priorities and make a meeting for each issue unless your boss requests that you submit multiple issues all at once. Think of this style of contact because bosses are more likely to be Linear in their approach than Analogue. They will be overwhelmed by a Big Picture approach so prevalent in a brainstyle with which they are less aware than their own. Breathe in and remember they are as vulnerable to overload as you are—it's just a different style of overload.

Fourth: In preparation, practice talking out what you want to say with someone else to see that your approach is orderly and understandable.

Fifth: Envision or role play yourself in the setting where you will meet.

Sixth: Develop notes of how you'll open the meeting.

Seventh: Expect small gains with your problem initially, not the whole world. Small increments will help you and the authority get used to facing the differences between you. The job may be done slowly, but the results become strong.

Eighth: Remember to breathe. Practice this daily in all sorts of environments. You'd be amazed how many of us hold our breath when we are working hard, which often means we have some fear rolling around inside of ourselves, often at a low, but persistent level, draining our energy.

And finally: when you're talking to your boss, say to yourself, "I am talking to my boss and I'm only focusing on him/her, what is being said, and how it seems to be feeling/looking." If you shift your attention to feeling afraid or worrying how the authority will respond, you'll lose track of what you want to achieve. Keep your focus on the authority. You may even say silently to yourself, "Listen." "What is being said?" "What does the authority seem to be feeling?" "How is the person responding?" There is nothing in the world more important to you than the person you're talking to and what he or she is saying and feeling. Try practicing this approach beforehand with a colleague or friend.

Choose extracurricular activities that you can practice in off hours such as yoga, Tai chi, and other systematic physical programs that can help you gain control over your body and psyche.

Perhaps you'd like to increase your focus of attention in situations you feel are important. Choose activities in which you have to stay focused to hit a ball or catch a pass. Maybe you need to meet a deadline and you set a timer so that you have a reminder when such and such a time is up. With practice, your memory is likely to adjust to that amount of time. Before long, you may find yourself speeding up in order to finish on time. Practice does help focus if you remain mindful and alert yourself that you are practicing to improve your attention. Choose an outlet that feels like a good fit for you. Honor your preferences.

While you are building your powerfulness, focus, and balance, believe in your own right to be. You will find an ally in belief—belief in yourself, belief that your way is the right way for you, your truth. Above all, believe in yourself.

Truth is one of the strongest, most powerful approaches to use when facing any situation. Believe in yourself, and no one can counter that. You can be told that what you are saying is wrong;

but if you believe that the way you see something is right for you, then it *is* Right for You.

Your feelings will tell you whether something is true. And if you feel afraid in a situation, listen to the fear, analyze your feelings, and I bet you'll figure out why you're afraid. Often we are trying to do something that we think we *ought* to be doing, but don't *want* to do or we're trying to do something that doesn't *fit* us.

I'll always remember when I had a talk show on KLIF Talk Radio in Dallas. I was recruited to represent the station in a Trivia Contest because I had the highest education level of anyone working there.

Upon hearing the news, my stomach immediately felt as if it had fallen from the top of a very tall building. You know the feeling. I would describe it as one of terror. I became so destabilized that I couldn't even answer the request right away. Finally, I bought time, saying, "I'll let you know tomorrow." To get grounded, I went for a walk in a lovely park after the show, I had a cup of coffee, and started to journal (journaling really helps me figure things out).

Slowly, I realized what the problem was. My physical body and emotional system figured out what my conscious mind hadn't realized. I felt that I was hovering over a dangerous abyss before I could realize what the problem was. I started to laugh and cry at the same time as I realized what was going on. Both were emotional releases as my thinking mind began to take over.

You see, I have a poor memory for details, facts, names, labels, etc. I can tell you how things work and what their functions are. I can tell you a story about them, but don't ask me their names.

If I entered the contest, I wouldn't be able to produce on the terms embraced by the contest. I felt that I would be letting both myself and my station down. That brought feelings of shame that I'd begun to experience before I realized what the problem was. I recalled all the times in school and even a few times early in my career when I'd been embarrassed, felt demeaned, and powerless in situations that I undertook because I thought I *should*.

I knew better than to put myself back into that kind of situation. I have both strengths and limitations because of my brainstyle, dyslexia, and learning differences. As a result, I had developed quite a case of Chronic Stress Response.

It had been necessary for me to identify my problems, then accept them, then become emotionally powerful enough to speak my truth about them and say "No," before I could harness my fears. By then though, I no longer felt "less than" because of these aspects of my makeup. At the same time, I was released to see a cadre of strengths, skills, and intelligence I had that others didn't have.

It's rather like a sumo wrestler who can't expect to win in an agility sport, but can win in a contest of strength. We all have what we have and it is just right for us. No one has all the abilities and skills and strengths or weaknesses of anyone else. So there is little to be afraid about.

Find your *fit*. Listen to your body's and mind's responses to anything that makes you feel afraid. As someone with ADD attributes, you will discover that you can trust what you feel—and if you feel afraid, pay attention. If you normally are comfortable walking on a street at night, fine. If suddenly you begin to feel prickles on the back of your neck and you start feeling afraid, pay attention, seek protection, and help.

I've discovered that people often tell me, "Oh, you 'shouldn't' do such and such. It's too dangerous." I quickly check my feelings about the situation. Then if I get an emotional green light, I say, "I appreciate your concern. I take really good care of myself, and I promise that if I feel anything amiss, I'll immediately take defensive action or abort what I was planning to do."

But if your fear reaches a phobic level, please do seek a mental health professional. You do not need to suffer. There are multiple ways to bring you relief including hypnosis (not the kind you see in old movies), medication, and desensitization techniques. But for the average situation you can learn to manage the type of fears so common to those of us with Chronic Stress Response and an ADD style of brain construction.

CLEARING GUILT: FORGIVING YOURSELF AND CHANGING VALUES

At first I thought that I would introduce you to CJ later on in this book. That was after my first interview with him. My, but he looked and seemed together. And for all intents and purposes he was—until I spent more time with him during a second interview. The shift in perspective opened a door that kept him from benefitting from the skills and talents that he was using as an ADD man who loves what he does and uses his ADD attributes for his success professionally. With an ADD Assessment Checklist rating that falls in the high range, CJ naturally discovered major useful ways to utilize his attributes for his success and enjoyment.

CJ was raised in a stable, mentally and behaviorally healthy family with a strong set of religious and social values consistently applied. An Armed Forces kid, he learned to adapt to all kinds of situations. The family was close-knit. He loved sports, was a naturally skilled athlete, and also benefited from the structure of training for and playing the sport. At first he was a player, and later a referee. He smiled with a twinkle in his eye as he said, "I liked the hardest games."

Throughout his life, he has kept physically fit and drug-free and only occasionally uses alcohol in moderation. Sports definitely supported outlets for his ADD attributes. The one down side that he has worked to change was that he had "quite a competitive temper." As a teen and young man, he told me that he would get very aggressive. But he has worked on moderating that and has not had a problem for years.

As a young adult, he learned to wield his emotional power in place of physical power when he chose to do so. Because he stayed in good shape, he still, in middle age, has considerable physical power.

CJ's choice of work has been "right on." Sales and marketing embraced him from the very beginning and has given him a fit for his brainstyle for years. He likes what he does for a living. A top-ranking salesman, he does what comes naturally. He has the innate ADD sensitivity and intuition that breeds opportunity. He reports that he "knows what others are thinking and feeling, and as a result, picks up on this and matches with the person easily in their relationship—a win-win outcome for salesman and client!"

Generally CJ works with a teammate who tends to keep track of the paperwork and details of their workflow. Over the years, interpersonal relationships with his various teammates have gone smoothly. There doesn't seem to be any question about the value of what he brings to the table. At sales meetings, he tends to have the ideas, sees the vision, and figures out how things need to function—for example, the flow of a marketing plan and the relationships between things, people, and projects. By doing his part, the whole team succeeds. The clients his firm services are top-notch, consistent quality sales outlets with successful businesses that know quality sales and marketing when they see it.

So, why isn't CJ totally at peace? It seems that since he was a school boy, he has had trouble paying attention in class. He reports that he still has the same trouble in business meetings. As we talked, it was evident that a large part of his problem is that he sees the overview quickly, figures out the process that is needed, rapidly sorts through suggestions made by others around the table, and knows how the whole meeting will work out. At that point, he becomes bored and his mind drifts. He begins to fidget and, to make matters worse, according to him, starts to crack jokes.

"I have a warped sense of humor. I hear something building that I think is funny, I blurt it out, get a belly laugh and crack everyone up. I feel like everyone says, 'Here comes fun CJ.'" And, that is not a good thing if the look on his face means anything. He truly does not see the value in how he is. His teammates apparently do, but not CJ. His teammates love his sense of humor, even the bosses. But he feels embarrassed at what comes out of his mouth—even though, in reality, it is tasteful and genuinely funny. Everyone is glad for the lighter mood and sees CJ as an asset.

On the road with other sales people and buyers with whom he meets, his relationship skills flourish and he and the others have "good times." It would seem that his humor did no harm and, if anything, increased the depth of long-lasting trust relationships with his clients and coworkers.

The second issue that bothers CJ is his memory. Starting in school, he remembers how hard it was for him to retain what was said. As with business, it was not a failure to remember what was being taught or what was going on, but was and continues to be in the area of remembering by rote: labels and names. He never forgets the way things function, the processes or relationships of how things work, or the patterns between things, people, and/or projects and goals.

In other words, his brain doesn't retain information communicated in a Linear mode, detail by detail, but does retain information communicated in an Analogue mode.

When I questioned him further about this and shared the differences created by brainstyles, he told me he was raised to believe that rote memory was critical and *the* way to be. That meant you were smart. No wonder he has a lowered sense of himself (the wounding) because of the simple difference between his style of brain and that heralded by the culture.

I asked him how he was so effective at accomplishing things, including keeping track of the necessary details, and he told me that he uses "cheat sheets" and writes on his hands so he can "read" the information that he may need when he's faced with having to speak about sales figures and the like.

"Does that work for you?" I asked.

"Yes, but I feel like I'm really cheating. I shouldn't be doing that. I feel jealous of the people who don't need to do it and can carry the numbers and information in their heads to be instantly called up. And I feel ashamed because I can't do that."

"Who cares?"

"No one, really. But I do."

My attempts to explain the differences of how people recall things did not break through the beliefs that he holds tightly.

In retrospect, CJ has all that it takes to be living a life that he actually likes in alignment with his *True Self*, using his talents to advantage. Corny as it may sound, he could be happy but, sadly, because of a belief system that is hard wired within him of the *right* way and the *not right* way to be, he feels guilty within himself. You would never know it in public because his facade is A-1.

CJ is trapped, wounded from an overly rigid value system based on early learning that fails to take into account brainstyle diversity. He doesn't need to make accommodations in his work life or personal life. He does need, for his mental health and self-esteem, to consider the truth of why he feels the way he does, which is not a problem socially or interpersonally, so that he doesn't feel guilty about his *True Self*'s makeup.

To do that, let us consider one method of changing our values as adults.

Changing Your Values

As an example of how to change a value, we will work with the belief, "You should have been able to do better in school." Then we'll use this method to decide if you want to keep that value or change it. And now it's your turn. If you feel even slightly guilty that you *should* have been able to do better in school, then use this method to decide if you want to keep that value or change it.

Consider the following questions and write your answers down or speak them to a partner. Remember, the value being considered is:

"You *should* have been able to do better in school."

Now ask yourself:

- Who did I learn that belief from in the first place? Maybe you find yourself thinking about how your parents and teachers always told you that you could do better if you'd just tried harder. Maybe they said, "You just need to pay more attention." Maybe you were judged as disordered, that is, maybe you learned something was *wrong* with you.
- Have I continued to believe that something is wrong with me because I am afraid I might be disapproved of if I change my belief about myself? (Notice who comes to mind as you think about this question.) Maybe you'll even feel afraid that others will argue with you or even laugh at you.
- What new information do I have now to consider that may change my original viewpoint? You now know a number of explanations that are new to you:
  - You know that there is a different way to look at ADD now than when you were a kid.
  - You know it is a diversity issue and that ADD is a normal brainstyle.
  - You know your brainstyle simply processes information differently than people with a non-ADD brainstyle.
  - In the past, teaching methods simply didn't *fit* you. Often they still don't, because this idea is new.
  - Presently, you have your own way to learn and do what fits you.

- ◦ And the way you are is important for the community at large because diversity brings balance.

- What are some of the side effects or costs of your old belief? Feelings of guilt and self-blame have probably caused you pain over the years. You may also have acted out your frustration and anger behaviorally. Perhaps you have a history of overeating, or drinking too much, or of losing your temper. Maybe your guilt is accompanied by feelings of depression because of the old belief.

- What new feelings do you have about your old *should* belief? Maybe you are beginning to realize that you did try as hard as you could, but you couldn't make things go well. You've never meant to do *wrong*. You're beginning to realize that you were, and even now may be, the victim of an incorrect belief that did not allow you to learn or find your *True Self*.

- You can now realize that your old *should* was incorrect and unworkable. Maybe you even have empathy for your inner child who survived a setting that didn't *fit*. You can now right a wrong helping your inner child and your current self.

Next, you can use the chart in figure 3.1 to help you update what you, the adult, now choose to believe. Look at the column on the left. It shows you how to keep the same value you were taught in childhood. Simply say to yourself, "I choose to keep the same value I had when I was young." You may want to add, "Now I understand why it was so hard for me. I no longer have to feel guilty and I can still believe what I believed then."

You've made a choice and now the adult you *owns* the value you currently live by, so you will no longer need to feel guilty.

If you feel that you would like to change your belief about your value, consider the column on the right side of the page. There, you'll find four steps to take to fully *own* the value.

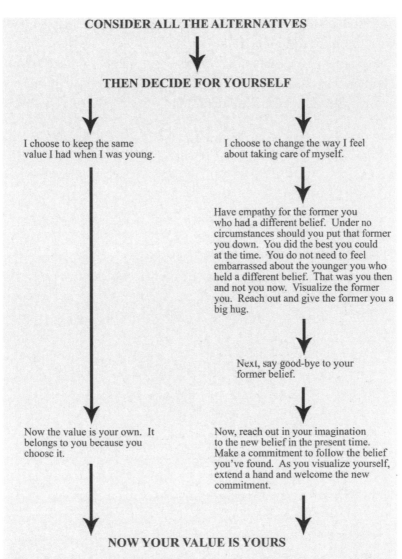

CONSIDER ALL THE ALTERNATIVES

THEN DECIDE FOR YOURSELF

I choose to keep the same value I had when I was young.

I choose to change the way I feel about taking care of myself.

Have empathy for the former you who had a different belief. Under no circumstances should you put that former you down. You did the best you could at the time. You do not need to feel embarrassed about the younger you who held a different belief. That was you then and not you now. Visualize the former you. Reach out and give the former you a big hug.

Next, say good-bye to your former belief.

Now the value is your own. It belongs to you because you choose it.

Now, reach out in your imagination to the new belief in the present time. Make a commitment to follow the belief you've found. As you visualize yourself, extend a hand and welcome the new commitment.

NOW YOUR VALUE IS YOURS

It doesn't matter what you decide. Your values are your business. What matters is that **you** choose them. It is important that you are conscious of what you believe and why you believe it. Then you can act accordingly, free of guilt and resentment.

Figure 3.1.

Do those steps now, either in writing, talking to a partner, or say them out loud to yourself.

Now your new perspective makes your value belong to you.

Either way you decide is fine for you. Congratulations—you now own the values by which you live.

4

THE DIFFERENT FACES OF ADD

By 1997, it was clear to me that ADD behavior and issues were situationally exacerbated by a lack of *fit* between our brainstyle and the tasks and situations with which we were confronted. But living near a small Texas town at the time gave me a liberal education in a whole new part of our American culture—the culture of small-town America populated by people who were born, raised, and remained in their birthplace environment their whole lives— and introduced me to many people who lived *well* with their ADD intact in settings where there were more quality opportunities that *fit* their brainstyle.

It also became clear to me that there are several different types, or faces, of the ADD brainstyle. We are even more than a community of people with diverse brainstyles; there is great diversity even within ADD. On table 4.1, you'll see a description of the three main types of ADD that unfolded for me as I interacted with more and more people with this wonderful brainstyle.

Living in the woods near Bastrop, Texas, also gave me the time to better study myself. What did I discover, having come to the

Table 4.1. Types and Characteristics of ADD

ADD General Characteristics

Traits:

Sees the big picture, thinks in terms of how things function, pays attention to patterns and relationships within the big picture, expresses high levels of activity (physical, mental, emotional, and verbal), learns by doing, has inner locus of perception and control, is responsive, has strong sensing capability, resonates to the rhythmic timing of nature.

Types:

These core ADD characteristics seem to surface in adults in three distinct ways shown below. People with ADD may fall into one of three categories, or they can exhibit a blend of two or all three types.

Type I
Outwardly Expressed ADD (ADHD), The Active Entertainer

Traits:

Outwardly active, spontaneous, high risk taker, wide mood capability, quick to change, reacts to external pressure, highly demonstrative, multi-tasks, expresses temper outwardly, prefers to break large tasks into segments creating many small tasks.

In Linear situations:

Easily bored, short attention span, dislikes long-term projects, becomes reactive, dislikes repetition, blames others when frustrated, expresses temper.

Type II
Inwardly Directed ADD, The Restless Dreamer

Traits:

Very empathetic, sticks to jobs liked, slow to change, very sensitive, visionary/dreamer, often highly creative, good problem solver, prefers freedom to explore, restless.

In Linear situations:

Tends to self-blame, distractible when bored, burns out, tends to depression, vacillates, tries too hard.

Type III
Highly Structured ADD, The Conscientious Controller

Traits:

Very organized, likes structure, has trouble self-structuring, perfectionistic, highly focused, talkative, dislikes interruptions, mentally restless, systematic problem solver, takes charge in a crisis, prefers to work a task from beginning to end without a break.

In Linear situations:

Demanding, rigid, judgmental, obsessively worries, loses temper, controlling.

awareness of just how ADD I am? Two distinct types of ADD influenced my body, mind, and spirit: Type I Outwardly Expressive ADD that "hit the road running" and Type II Inwardly Directed that thought about everything that was happening to me and around me, wrote poetry, talked to the animals, and socialized as I leaned on the back of my pickup truck. In this way, I became immersed in the culture of the town. What a new experience, having always lived in cities.

The sensitive, kinesthetic part of me was happy living and learning in this laid-back environment, while professional demands filled me with "booming, buzzing, confusion" as I organized, or tried to organize my travels, writing, and personal life.

Funny thing about the subsequent implications of these experiences is the way in which they are showing up now as, sixteen years later, I am reviewing what is important to share with you so you gain a well-rounded picture of ADD in the early twenty-first century.

As I progress with sharing the Different Faces of ADD, I find myself embracing the wonderful gifts ADD brings me as a fifty/fifty Mixed Type I and Type II ADD woman. And I remember the same "lessons" I am sharing with you: that I may fully live and relive my way of functioning even when it is dreadfully hard, for my perspective shows me who I am and what I have to offer others with what tumbles out of this ADD woman called Lynn.

There are many more faces I want to share with you, so that you can get an idea of the diversity attributed to ADD. We'll start with Belinda—nicknamed Belle, as in "Belle of the Ball"—who's classic Type I ADHD. Next comes Jai, Type II ADD without hyperactivity. Next, you can read about the seeding of a Type III Highly Structured ADD category as it unfolds with Quentin's story. He's followed by Roderick, Max, and Joe. Finally in this section you'll experience stories of people who appear to have Mixed Types of ADD, people like Scotty and Olivia. Many of us are a mixture of ADD types. We definitely are a community of diversity in many ways.

As you read through the stories in this section, I'd suggest you pay attention to how you relate to each person. Whether you're male or female doesn't matter. You'll find that you relate to the person and his or her experiences, get a sense of familiarity as you read about the person—or you'll find that you do not relate to them and their experiences.

As you read the stories of our fellow travelers, I suggest you ask yourself, "Could this be me?" Let the sense of like-kind roll around in your mind and check your gut-level feelings. Then consider whether you are a lot, some, or very little like the person. In this way you'll be doing your own diagnostics toward discovering how the puzzle called You is made.

Of course you'll come out with your own unique patterns, blends, and talents within your general brain construction—a construction that will be perfect for You. You'll find through others' stories another someone to relate to as you begin your ADD journey.

Finally, you'll find questions at the end of each section that can help you compare their story to yours.

TYPE I: ADD WITH HYPERACTIVITY (ADHD)

Belle (Belinda)

"You Saved my Life! I'm ADD off the wall!" Belle says, catching my attention with her exclamations.

It wasn't that long ago when, if we thought of ADD, we were really visualizing ADD in action: big, bold, expressive, active, and unignorable.

Enter Belle, the five-year-old darling, singing and dancing her way around a Texas dance hall in San Antonio, delighting even the most somber elders and giggly teenagers who mostly ignored little kids. Not Belle. Everyone loved a Belle.

Talk about embracing life. Belle was the poster child of ADD in 1971 before ADD was even invented as a disorder linked to mental disorders and completely misunderstood for what it was and can be.

Belle's mama always told her that she was special, treating her like someone who had charisma, enthusiasm, and great people skills. Mama said she would help Belle do whatever she was supposed to do in life.

By age eight, she got her first guitar at Christmas. But her enthusiasm quickly dampened when her first teacher, a professional jazz musician, had her plucking one note at a time while trying to teach music theory to her. As she summed it up, "It wasn't going to happen, not for this kid who wanted to sing and play the guitar right away." Translated, it meant, "a Linear approach to teaching music wasn't going to happen for this seriously Analogue/kinesthetic learner."

School had its ups and downs, too. Belle, described it well in our interview: "My sixth grade teacher brought my reading level up from fourth grade to eighth grade the year I was with her." After a moment's hesitation, Belle added with a sweet smile, "She saw the twinkle in my eye, though I was an average student."

Using music as the focal point of her middle school and high school years, Belle continued to feel good about herself. Her eighth grade choir teacher asked her to sing a solo for the fall concert. The opportunity led to her entertaining the choir class for the last fifteen minutes every Friday. With a smile in her eyes, Belle added, "And I sang my way through many book reports during high school, too. I loved this, but it didn't endear me to my classmates. I began to feel very alone as a teen."

Around that time, her mama "hooked me up with a new music teacher who taught me what I wanted to know in a way that

I could manage. For example, he started with chords, not single notes. Then he also taught me whole songs that I wanted to sing. And he encouraged my song writing and taught me how to develop a song. From these beginnings, I was interested enough to learn single notes and music theory."

This reminds me of my ADD son's experience in elementary school. He was enthusiastic about playing the drums. The music teacher said he had to learn to play bells first and wouldn't let him play any kind of drum. So he quit.

A lot of Nonlinear kids simply cannot start at one note and move on from there in a sequential, linear, straight line. They have to follow their feelings, making a sound design or picture of rhythms or some pattern circulating in their heads. Eventually they'll embrace most or all of the elements involved in the acquisition of the playing of the total instrument, creating their own symphony.

In Belle's case, the most important motivation of all was her liking for her teacher who believed in her. His ability to communicate that belief was like hooking the ring on the merry-go-round.

At fifteen, Belle's mama recorded four of her daughter's original songs on her own country album—four songs that her guitar teacher had helped her write. In the same year of 1982, Belle heard her songs on the radio for the very first time and learned how much her mama and others valued her talent.

At seventeen, when Belle received several calls from her Sunday school teacher about missing Sunday school, she began to take more responsibility for the important things that she valued, especially her church connection. Solo club and restaurant gigs on Saturday nights gave way to early rising on Sunday morning. As she became responsible for her more mature values, her ADD paid off. Her Sunday school teacher said she'd help Belle in any way, if she would finish a gospel song she'd failed to finish. Belle did finish it and the teacher did help her from inspiration to financial support. She aided Belle with her music ministry—a ministry from her heart.

At one point, the reality of Belle's obvious Type I ADD helped her avoid a job she didn't like as a church administrator. Her supervisor agreed that filing was not her strength. Instead she worked with the youth director, led the youth choir, and got her first church singing gig while going to college off and on. It took her seven years to graduate, but she finished.

In time, Belle learned to adapt her innate skills to the big world. The first goal became one of survival. Next came proficiency in using her ADD skills to express her *True Self*. Finally, she learned to attend to the making of ADD accommodations to the Linear requirements that are necessary for daily living—things like schedules, bookkeeping, and constructing walls to protect her sensitivity and outlets for her creativity.

Gently, the balance that adult living requires was coming under her control. She had made the grade, ADD and all. Belle knew who she was as she entered adulthood, having received a lot of support along the way using her natural talents and gifts.

But then the fairyland *fit* of Belle's youth took a downward turn when she left home from San Antonio at the age of thirty-three with her husband who had decided to change careers. They moved to a tiny town and ran head first into a cultural wall that didn't *fit* Belle's personality or style. Nor did her brainstyle *fit*. The structure that Belle's mother provided for her was seriously shaken—a belief and structure that so perfectly supported and maintained Belle in her early years that when they were gone at the same time, she felt lost.

You see, Belle's mother died at the same time, leaving her without having built and strengthened her own coping muscles. It seems that the daughter's belief in herself died when her mother died.

Similar to Henry's experience (chapter 2, p. 71), Belle's too-good fit in childhood did not allow her the opportunity to learn to cope with the Linear world that is unavoidable as we grow up. At the critical young adult time when each of us is finding ways to discover and adapt our budding *True Selves* for living in the world at large, we need more mentorship and support rather than less.

Unfortunately, the desire to "do it" ourselves, to prove ourselves, is often strong at the same time. But, also unfortunately, our inexperience is mighty in accommodating our ADD skills for life in the world at large—a world that requires a lot of Linear skills and takes time and learning that is not natural to us.

You and Belle: Type I, Outwardly Expressive ADD

Think about yourself as you mark the Type I ADD traits shown on table 4.2.

Table 4.2. Type I, Outwardly Expressive ADD/ADHD and You

Think about yourself as you mark the following traits in relation to you. If you demonstrated a trait in childhood, mark it with a "c," even if you've learned to control the trait as you've grown up. Follow the "c" with either "H" for high, "S" for some, and "L" for low. (See table 4.1 for additional ADD characteristics.)

Trait	Exhibited in Childhood	High	Some	Low
Outwardly Active				
Outwardly Expressive				
Wide Mood Swings				
Highly Demonstrative				
Rejects External Pressure				
Multi-Tasks				
Expresses Temper Outwardly				
Quick to Change				
Easily Bored				
Short Attention Span				
Becomes Reactive				
Blames Others When Frustrated				
Prefers to Break Tasks Into Segments				

After filling out the table, you might want to journal or discuss about Type I ADD. How did reading about Belle affect you? How did Belle's story make you feel? How did seeing the traits listed in table 4.2 make you feel?

TYPE II: ADD WITHOUT HYPERACTIVITY

Jai

As long ago as the late 1980s, I began to notice that not everyone who was having difficulties with learning, organization, and thinking about and following through on tasks was hyperactive. I suppose because hyperactivity is so obvious, it was easy in the beginning to think ADD was defined exclusively with hyperactivity as a part of the syndrome.

Soon, however, I discovered that a few other professionals also were questioning whether all people with ADD were hyperactive.

My big step came when I met Jai. My awareness of a second type of ADD began to unfold in my office one day in the late 1980s when Jai, an intelligent, well-educated (computer science degree) business owner, came for a consultation. Despite being raised in a strong family, having received a good education, marrying a loving and active woman, and being given support in establishing his own business, Jai was not succeeding up to potential that he or others expected. Personality-wise, he was quiet, a bit aloof, and inattentive to social cues. But he spoke clearly as he began our interview.

Sharing that he had wanted to become self-employed because he had a lot of ideas that he felt he could turn into marketable programs and successful business ventures, he'd somehow not been able to bring these ideas and dreams to fruition. This made him feel depressed and fed feelings of low self-esteem. He just didn't understand what he was doing wrong. He simply didn't seem to have what it takes to be a self-employed entrepreneur.

At home, his low-keyed nature bothered his wife. With her own professional job, which she'd scaled back to part time once their first two children were born, she wanted more help with the running of their daily lives.

No mention of ADD occurred at this first meeting. Background in place, it was agreed that he and his wife would return for joint consultation in a few days.

Initially, we worked with typical marriage counseling information-gathering, problem-solving, and skill-building. Jai and his wife pretty much told the same story and held similar values. Both were frustrated, both tired, and yet they both loved each other and their children and wanted to keep their family intact. Both seemed mentally healthy and devoid of the bad habits or character disorders that can seriously compromise a marriage.

One day, unclear about the origins feeding their problems, I had Jai come in for individual counseling. As we talked, I began to notice something that I'd not noticed when he and his wife were together.

Sitting opposite him, in close proximity with no distractions, I saw a nonstop series of slowly unfolding movements. He'd brush his forehead, then cross one leg over the other. After a short while, he'd shift his seating position so that his legs were reversed. Then he'd bend one foot upward, stretching his ankle, followed by circling his foot clockwise, and so on.

Sloth speed is faster than Jai's movements. Though barely noticeable, this nonintrusive movement was constant and regular. He surely didn't fit the image of what one might expect from an ADD brainstyle.

The moment I realized that Jai's activity style might just explain his problems if I considered ADD without hyperactivity, new insights and interventions fell into place. He sat quietly while I was considering my next move. I decided to ask Jai what he was thinking.

He said, "Oh, not really anything."

When I responded, "You know, I'd really like to know," he started talking about the business, some of his technical ideas, his dreams, and then his family.

In turn I asked another question, "Does your mind think a lot?"

As I'd guessed by then, his answer was, "All the time."

Ah, there it was—his ADD was mental. His temperament was quiet.

At the next session, we talked about his work and got on the subject of organization, time management, and goal completion. I realized that his lack of ability to organize in a Linear way, a skill necessary to administrate a business, explained why he was not able to apply his technological skills for use toward a goal.

Jai would have to learn over time to organize. The best way for him or anyone with Analogue processing to learn would be by using the apprenticeship model. So he'd need someone else to do the organizing. Through repetition, he could watch, listen, learn, and help to do what the other person designed. Little by little, he would learn the Linear process and be able to take more and more of the responsibility to plan and implement it.

Likely, it would be more efficient for him to always have much of the planning and structuring turned over to someone else, because it would always take more energy for him to perform the job since the Linear way is simply not his innate strength. But he would be able to keep abreast of the plans and programs and more easily and effectively add his input, his creativity, and his skill base to the business.

It was apparent that his high level of awareness fed his low self-esteem as he saw that he was not producing up to par—a par set both by the values held by his current family as well as his parental family and most importantly, by himself. No wonder he was nearly paralyzed.

We spent several sessions talking about ADD, and his wife, Monica, joined us. It seemed she had strong organizational and management skills as well as an outgoing personality that helped her "get things done." She didn't like being still, but rather preferred to be on the move—though at this time her energy was directed toward trying to get Jai on the move, since he was viewed as the family's major wage earner.

It became apparent that Monica was what I later came to call a "Bridge Person," that is, someone with both Analogue and Linear skills.

Coming to that conclusion, our next step was to explore the personal family aspects of their relationship. They chose to begin by bringing up areas in the marriage in which Jai did not live up to his wife's expectations. And we looked at areas of expectation that overwhelmed him.

Follow-through and time management were high on the list, as when he failed to remember to order tickets for an evening out, or to pick up dry cleaning on the way home from work, or pay the car insurance on time. His deficits were little things, but extremely annoying over the long haul. On the other hand, he was great with the kids and loved to cook.

Restless, he didn't want to go to bed when his wife did—a trait that she took personally. And he'd never been able to figure out how to tell her that her stroking his arm or back drove him crazy. Ah, ADD sensitivity does have a down side, at least until couples figure out how to work around it to advantage.

Also, I discovered that he was a marathon runner. It seems that the only time he really relaxed was when he ran until he experienced the runner's high. Running helped him sleep, helped his mind slow down, and helped his mood become mellow. Unfortunately, Monica wanted to go to bed soon after the children because she was an early riser and tired at night. Immediately they began to talk about ways to handle the timing of their personal intimacy.

The really good news was that once ADD was out of the proverbial bag, solutions began to tumble forth. Small changes made all the difference in the world. Holding replaced stroking. He talked about his need to slow down his mind in order to be able to give his wife the personal attention she deserved and desired, so she knew not to take his needs personally. They felt they could work out their differences.

Because Jai had been chronically depressed for as long as he could remember, I was able to work with his primary-care physician to find a medication that treated his depression in order to buy time for him to develop skill-based interventions to accommodate his Inwardly Directed ADD.

Larger changes followed. As he expanded his repertoire of coping skills aided by medication, Jai was able to manage details better, partner with colleagues in the workplace, and trade jobs with his wife at home. He took over preparation for weekend meals, and began to pick up the kids after school and work with them on homework, after which he often cooked dinner. Meanwhile, Monica handled their finances and household business, dealing with detailed organization and planning.

As a couple, they learned to work from a position of their strengths, with Jai taking the kids to their activities while his wife did the scheduling and recording of reminders. Oh, and by the way, this came in very handy a couple of years later when they had triplets who required lots and lots of attention and scheduling.

Jai learned a much-needed lesson: none of us can do all things. But we can be a happy, successful member of a team that helps others as well as ourselves. Once we learn to accept ourselves as we are innately constructed, no longer try to hide what we can't do, and communicate what we can do, we make a good partner. Teamwork is a powerful tool in all relationships.

After the breakthrough with Jai, I began to notice many people who had jobs as teachers, counselors, and childcare workers who also did not have obvious hyperactivity, but did have a "silent" type of ADD that at first went unrecognized. I saw mechanics and trades people who used their gentler form of activity to advantage—as long as they didn't have to sit at a desk all day. By moving around, the physical restlessness of their ADD was an asset on the job. The kinesthetic style of their hands-on work focused their mental activity toward a tangible goal that was satisfying.

Only as their difficulties surfaced—with unaccommodated organization, attention to mental details whizzing around without a physical outlet, hypersensitivity, and the need to learn kinesthetically rather than "about" a subject—did it become apparent that ADD was not the only kid on the block.

Just as activity level and expressive behavior reflected Type I ADD, restlessness, sensitivity, and high creativity reflected Type II ADD. Depression is substituted for outwardly focused aggression under stress. Both groups simply need to learn to utilize their assets and curb their vulnerability.

You and Jai: Type II Inwardly Directed ADD

Think about yourself as you consider the traits of Type II Inwardly Directed ADD shown in table 4.3. and mark the traits in relation to you.

After considering the traits in the table, you might want to journal or discuss about Jai and yourself. How do you relate to Jai and how are you different? How did reading about Jai affect you? How did Jai's story make you feel?

MY FIRST GLIMPSE OF TYPE III ADD

Quentin, Roderick, Max, and Joe

Back in 1997, I didn't realize that I was seeing yet another type of ADD, one that would resurface into my conscious awareness several years later.

Quentin's coming to see me because he was restless and depressed led me to realize there might be another form of ADD: a Type III. He wanted to be evaluated for ADD because he'd heard me talking about the traits and he identified with a num-

Table 4.3. Type II, Inwardly Directed ADD and You

Think about yourself as you mark the following traits in relation to you. If you demonstrated a trait in childhood, mark it with a "c," even if you've learned to control the trait as you've grown up. Follow the "c" with either "H" for high, "S" for some, and "L" for low. (See table 4.1 for additional ADD characteristics.)

Trait	Exhibited in Childhood	High	Some	Low
Inwardly Active				
Inwardly Expressive				
Very Sensitive				
Very Empathic				
Sticks to Job Liked				
Visionary/Dreamer				
Often Highly Creative				
Slow to Change				
Good Problem Solver				
Hands-On Learner				
Restless				
Prefers Freedom to Explore				
Expresses Anger as Depression				
Empathetic				

ber of them. A self-employed landscape gardener, he specialized in building rock gardens with fountains and exotic pools, water plants, lotus blossoms, fish, and decorative sculptures. He absolutely loved what he did and made good money working at his own pace. He liked keeping his own hours, being outdoors, and having the power to choose the jobs he wanted.

His biggest complaint was that he was having problems with billing and recordkeeping. The woman who had helped him for years had recently moved away when her husband retired. Her leaving immediately left him feeling lost, devastated, and very, very anxious.

In trying to explain how he felt, he told me a story I've never forgotten, a story about ADD. Pretending to use a deck of playing cards, he pretended to carefully build a structure made with them. When he attempted to put a top card on his building, he said, "It's like I live in a house of cards that I've built with my own hands—just like this one. Then I have to start over again, building from the ground up . . . over and over again."

Thinking about Quentin's example, I realized he no longer had a structure to support him since his office assistant left. It was his inability to create a structure that was undermining his well-being. He felt overwhelmed because he didn't have the skills to keep track of the details that were necessary for his artistry to pay off.

His problem isn't much different from a highly skilled accountant who is unable to draw a satisfactory clientele because, as a shy person, she doesn't have the communication skills and charisma to attract business, or to network and act in a gregarious manner because of her brainstyle diversity. Again, individuals rarely have a full complement of Linear and Analogue skills.

Quentin, like Jai, reinforced the meaning of teaming to protect his talents so he could build a strong business in order to make a good living. By compensating for the business demands he couldn't fulfill by finding a replacement for the administrative assistant who left, Quentin could again do what he did well.

In the long run, Quentin made more money spending money than he could make alone. Hiring or teaming with someone paid off. Oh yes, and subsequent to finding a new office manager, his depression went away.

I didn't know after my interview with Quentin whether he only reflected variations of Type II ADD people or if, in fact, there was another form of ADD that might be mixed in with the Type II. It's less important to "prove" that there is a Type III than to fashion an accommodation that helps people live and work smoothly with their ADD style of brain construction.

He seemed to have problems with self-structuring. His experiences sowed a seed that stayed in the back of my mind. Later that year, however, I observed in one week's time a set of experiences that led me to realize that by postulating an additional form of

ADD, Type III, a person could gain understanding that would lead to more effective use of his or her brainstyle.

It all began early one week when I saw a happily married middle-aged couple in my private practice. The husband, Roderick, had recently retired from the Armed Forces. His wife, Georgia, and he had been looking forward to their new life. He was eager to spend time enjoying activities that he'd not had time for during much of his adult life. Jointly, they planned to travel and camp together, visit their adult children and grandchildren, and tackle building projects around the house as well as take up dancing again after many years.

Though their dreams were still in place and they continued to care deeply for one another, something had gone awry. Both husband and wife told the same story. It seems at first that Roderick enthusiastically talked about his dreams, the many things he wanted to try, and was even eager to get at the fix-it projects that had been waiting for him, some for years.

But it didn't take long before Roderick discovered that days simply raced by without his accomplishing much. At first he didn't worry because he figured he simply wanted to enjoy free time and loved the idea of sleeping late—except the sleeping late part didn't last more than a week. Then he began to feel bored with "nothing to do." His free time began to weigh on him. Guilt tracked him down as he simply didn't seem to get anything done.

Georgia didn't want to intrude or press him, though she had eagerly awaited their "new life." Soon, she, too, was getting restless with the "I'm a gunna" routine. Yes, he was "wasting his time." One day, she asked if there was anything she could do to help him get started and, for the first time, he raised his voice —something he'd rarely, if ever, done, gruffly answering, "No." After this "minor blow-up," they decided they'd better get some help.

I'm not sure what led me to the questions I asked the day they came in for their one-and-only counseling visit, but they led us to a solution for implementing their new life. Basically, what occurred to me was that Roderick did really well in the Armed Forces where there is a rigid structure that directed what he and everyone else did. He excelled in that setting, working efficiently and effortlessly most of the time. And he liked the environment and his high level of productivity. When he returned home full time, he walked into a situation where there was no structure for the things he wanted to do.

He understood the implication as we talked further. He realized that the much-sought freedom he cherished and had looked forward to for so long carried the need to be able to structure time and jobs in order to make them work. But the look on his face as he said this conveyed the painful awareness that he didn't have a clue how to start to self-structure.

As we uncovered what was really going on, including his ownership of a lack of skills needed to build an activity structure, it became apparent that he needed help to create a plan to his and his wife's liking. At that point Roderick looked at his wife with a shy smile and she returned it with a broad grin. You see, she's the one who had run the household for years, kept track of the finances, and was a naturally skilled plan maker and implementer. She even liked doing these things.

She had felt willing, even eager to take over the job to structure their new life, but hadn't wanted to override her husband or intrude on his plans to do what he wanted to do. Now that the truth was out, they easily agreed to divide the "chores." Georgia would develop a structure that worked for both of them. Roderick could give input any time, though he rarely did. And they would work together to implement their plans.

I did not see them again, but from time to time I would receive a letter or pictures showing me their travels and adventures as they enjoyed life together.

Later that week, I saw Max and Joe, two airline pilots who had been with an airline company that was downsizing. These older pilots with seniority had been offered buy-out packages if they retired early. And both were experiencing a terrible time, as Roderick had, trying to learn to manage time in their newly freed-up, unstructured lives.

It would take time but, with awareness of their need to receive help with structuring their new lives, they had to find new interests that carried ready-made structures with them. They also had to deal with a tendency to hyper-focus, which made it hard on their spouses. Max's marriage made it with continued help and management of his ADD traits, but Joe's did not. Joe blamed his wife and family and the airline for his angry, anxious feelings and became obsessively over-controlling once he no longer had an airplane and crew to control.

You and Quentin, Roderick, Max, and Joe: Type III Highly Structured ADD

Think about yourself as you mark the traits of Type III Highly Structured ADD on table 4.4.

How did you relate to the stories of Quentin, Roderick, Max, and Joe? Did you get a sense of familiarity with them? Was it like finding "like-kind?" How do you differ from them?

How did reading about the four scenarios affect you? How did their stories make you feel?

MIXED TYPES OF ADD

You've just had a chance to get to know several people who primarily demonstrate a single type of ADD:

Type I ADD: Outwardly Expressed ADD, The Active Entertainer

Type II ADD: Inwardly Directed ADD, The Restless Dreamer

Type III ADD: Highly Structured ADD, The Conscientious Controller

Table 4.4. Type III, Highly Structured ADD and You

Think about yourself as you mark the following traits in relation to you. If you demonstrated a trait in childhood, mark it with a "c," even if you've learned to control the trait as you've grown up. Follow the "c" with either "H" for high, "S" for some, and "L" for low. (See table 4.1 for additional ADD characteristics.)

Trait	Exhibited in Childhood	High	Some	Low
Very Organized				
Likes/Needs Structure				
Expresses Anger Loudly				
Perfectionistic				
Highly Focused				
Talkative				
Likes Planning				
Dislikes Interruptions				
Mentally Restless				
Systematic Problem Solver				
Prefers Freedom to Explore				
Prefers to Work a Task from Beginning to End with No Break				

But many of us have a mixture of types, either two or three. The balance of the types can be equal or not. But, it behooves each of us to know about the balance so we are kind to ourselves as we find our place in the world around us. Even when a trait plays a minor role in our lives, we do not want to ignore it.

Scotty's Story, Mixed Types I and II

Scotty had earned a technical degree as an aircraft mechanic after high school. With a couple of years of hands-on experience, he felt comfortable in most work situations. If he didn't know how to fix something, he would tinker on his own until he understood how things worked. He also discovered he had a talent for designing new ways to accomplish old tasks, making them more efficient, and inventing techniques that no one had come up with before.

He loved his job. He most definitely hadn't loved school, and he never dreamed that he would love his work. Suddenly, he realized that he was "smart." What a change he felt with that awareness. For the first time in his life, he valued his skills. He felt his self-worth.

What Scotty hadn't realized was that he simply had a primarily Nonlinear style of brain construction that works differently than the style that is valued in school, a style that hadn't fit him well as he tried to learn in school.

Scotty and I crossed paths after he had become depressed because he'd been promoted at work. Prior to his promotion, he had been an on-call emergency electronic/mechanical specialist who was contacted when there was a difficult situation that needed immediate continual attention until the problem was fixed.

He loved working the intense, high-energy thirty-six-hour shifts, after which he was given three days off to recuperate and enjoy himself. He discovered he liked the intensity of the excitement he felt when he was called to gather his tools to head off to another urgent situation where time translated into money lost for the airline. And he loved getting extra recuperative time off to go home and work in his own shop designing and building all sorts of things: mobile devices for handicapped kids, and games and toys for sick kids so they could have more fun. Granted his age limit for "kids" went up to the grandparent generation. That's the kind of person he was.

But because he'd done so well on the job, his boss decided to promote him to management where he could earn more money. His promotion put him in charge of supervising and training other mechanics as well as become a part of the planning and development team. He also was expected to write reports of emergency situations so the staff could learn from what went wrong, how to correct it, and how to avoid it happening again. After all, he, more than anyone else, knew how to analyze the problems.

Scotty didn't much like the idea of moving into management, though he appreciated the opportunity, but he figured he should try it because his boss asked him to. Maybe he'd be okay making more money at a regular forty-hour-a-week job.

Unfortunately, Scotty hated management: not the people, but what they and he had to do to earn their pay. He simply disliked the job. He didn't like dressing up. He felt he was trapped, like being back in school. Nothing of interest ever happened, and having five days a week filled with work that he hadn't done well in the first place was bad. He felt as if he was never finished and he simply couldn't sit at a desk all day long. Trapped! is what he felt. Depressed! is what he became. And, to boot, there was no excitement about his job anymore.

Scotty decided to quit.

His boss wouldn't let him quit and gave him back his old job, but didn't understand why Scotty wouldn't want to progress.

Scotty didn't understand either until he learned about being a Mixed Type I and II ADD person who needed both activity and excitement at work while accomplishing his trade using hands-on skills that were natural to his Type II brainstyle. Both aspects of himself felt good when doing something extraordinary in the workforce that few others could do. Finally he felt he had value—unlike in school when he didn't feel proud of himself and his talents.

At the same time, his hobby reflected his feeling of empathy for others as he did things for people less fortunate. It made his sensitive heart and soul feel very, very good. He recognized immediately what fit his brainstyle, promising himself that he would live in a way that made him happy. He no longer felt "less than" other people.

And Scotty knew he was a valuable member of society. Neither job status nor money can provide what he felt when he worked at things that truly *fit* him. By following the guidelines that his *True Self* desired in order to be who he was meant to be, Scotty's self-esteem had recovered as he lived out his *True Self*. So can yours.

You and Scotty, Mixed Types I and II

Now take a look back at table 4.2 (Type I, Outwardly Expressive ADD/ADHD and You) and table 4.3 (Type II, Inwardly Directed ADD and You). When you look at the traits you've marked, have you identified a similar number on each table? How did you relate to Scotty and his story? Did you get a sense of familiarity with him? Was it like finding "like-kind?" How do you differ from Scotty? How did reading about Scotty affect you? How did Scotty's story make you feel?

Olivia's Story, Mixed Types II and III

After writing about meeting with Quentin, I decided that Olivia's story would give another dimension on Type II and Type III ADD. Rather quiet and shy, Olivia decided to take a job working out of her house doing telecommunications. In part it was a decision made after she had been evaluated for ADD. The evaluation showed her to be ADD without hyperactivity.

She knew she didn't like to socialize in large groups, the way it seemed everyone else at her last job liked to do. The new job *fit* her personal desires to forgo driving to work, allowed her to set her own work schedule, and potentially paid more than she'd previously made with less expense in the long run. So she decided to try the new job and settled into working from her home, which was near the office where I met with ADD support and training groups.

Olivia's visit to my office was prompted by a problem she'd not foreseen. Apparently everything was going well until she realized that she was "giving" herself too much break time, so that she either ran late at the end of the day or ran short on the amount of time that she had budgeted to work to meet her financial needs.

In answer to my question, "What do you do during break time?" she responded, "I get up, stretch, take a snack into the living room, and read a chapter out of whatever book I'm presently interested in. I figured one chapter would set a limit for me so that I wouldn't get lost in the story and spend too much time away from work during break."

"How's it working?"

"I was doing okay with the first two books. But then I started a third. It turned out that when I changed books, I read too long at lunch break. I'd felt really proud of myself until this happened. And I even reminded myself to be careful so I wouldn't read too long. I've always had trouble with time, but I have been better since working at home. So I figured that I'd finally gotten control over time because I'd made a commitment to myself."

Upset because of feeling like a failure, a few big tears ran down Olivia's face. "I don't know why I'm not being responsible. What's wrong with me?"

"Olivia, there's nothing seriously wrong with you—but like a lot of people who have an ADD style of brain construction, you can lose track of time when you're doing something that you really love. And, yes, you're trying hard, and you're a responsible person. But I bet you become a part of the story you're reading and, being kinesthetic, you forget what else is going on around you.

"How about my giving you a couple of tricks that ought to solve the problem so you can read at break time and also honor the commitments you make?"

Eagerly, Olivia agreed.

"How many pages were in the last book you were reading when you went over time?"

There was silence in the room for nearly a minute with a frown deepening on her face.

"Gosh, I don't know. But I think the chapters were pretty long."

"How long?" I asked softly, because I could tell she'd figured out the problem and didn't need me to jar her into awareness or rub in the point that she'd missed earlier.

"I don't really know," she sighed.

"Would you agree the chapters were probably longer than in the first book?

"Yes."

"All right, here's what I think happened. You were measuring your break by the time it took you to read a chapter. But when the chapter length increased, you were so absorbed in the story that another part of your mind didn't compute the amount of time you'd already used up. You hadn't been computing time, but chapters.

"In relation to your work time, you schooled yourself to sit down to work at a particular time and it didn't hurt anything if you got totally absorbed in it. Remember your motivation was very high 'on the job' because you wanted to work at home. True you will have a desire to stop break time on time, but the motivation is removed another step from being at your desk.

"Granted, some people seem to have an internal time sensor that keeps track of time, but lots of people don't. And besides, if you're measuring chapters, your sensor won't work properly. So you need to measure time. What ideas do you have to do that?"

"Well, if I promise to look up at the clock, I probably will get absorbed in the story and forget to do it. I need something that will get my attention. Oh, I have a kitchen timer that I can set."

"Great idea. How long do you want to read?"

"I think fifteen minutes is fine."

"I'd like to suggest that no matter where you are in the book, you must close it immediately when the timer goes off—because if you don't, you'll forget it rang. That's the way it happens for most of us ADD folks. I can't tell you how many pots I've burned up when I was typing at my computer and just wanted to finish a sentence after my timer went off. I've learned, no matter what, follow through at the moment the timer goes off, or else!"

Olivia laughed and agreed to give it a try.

In her final reporting visit, she brought me a lovely handmade bookmark similar to the ones she'd begun to make as a reward to herself for following through on her assignment. She was grateful that she had been able to solve her problem.

I heard several years later that she was still working out of her house, making good money, and enjoying her books. Kudos, Olivia!

You and Olivia, Mixed Types II and III

Think about yourself as you look back at the traits you marked in table 4.3 (Type II, Inwardly Directed ADD and You) and table 4.4 (Type III, Highly Structured ADD and You). Did you mark about the same number of traits on each table? How did you relate to Olivia when you read her story? Did you get a sense of familiarity? Was it like finding "like-kind?"

How do you differ from Olivia?

5

FINDING, DEALING WITH, AND GROWING THE *TRUE YOU*

For purposes of Embracing ADD—or any other brainstyle as a matter of fact—what you need to know about yourself is all tied up in the *True You*. But, what is this "thing," this "part" of us with which we are born? It is the core of everything we do. But, what does that mean?

Each of us may describe it differently, each in our own way. It's the engine and energy behind our behavior, feelings, and actions as well as our likes and dislikes. It is the source of our happiness. To be sure, some of us may have a grand and wonderful talent or skill, something that was apparent to others even as our two- to three-year-old selves began to be expressive. But even such a talent may not be your *True Self*—and you don't need an observable talent or skill to lead you to your *True You*.

Now that you're old enough, you can begin to actively seek the *True You*. Even if you are already using a talent seen in your childhood, you'll need to rediscover the part you now want to give attention to by growing your *True You* further. Even if you've never had a thought about who you are meant to be, you can begin now and follow the stories and practices that will let you find the wonderful feeling of belonging to yourself.

The *True You* is a sense of living and working the way that feels right to you. It is not the way you *think* you should live. It is not what your parents taught that you *ought* to be. It is not what the education system gave you good grades for or insisted that you spend endless hours pursuing. It is not necessarily a job track that you pursued as a young adult in order to make a living.

It is what makes you smile at yourself and others. It's what gives you a warm feeling in your solar plexus. It's what you feel like bragging about to yourself and others. It's what makes you eager to get up and sometimes makes your heart sing. It's what makes you grieve if something happens to interrupt your ability to use it.

It may stay the same during your whole adult life. On the other hand, your *True You* may be variegated with different interweaving interests and expressions. You may even find that you have several parts that are not particularly connected, but each has had its own time, drawing you to express it until you sensed that it was time to change direction or build a new style of expression with a newly evolved *True You*.

HOW DO YOU FIND AND BUILD YOUR *TRUE YOU?*

With all these variations of *True You* patterns and styles, how do you know how you are made? There are not eight or twelve variations or . . . It doesn't matter how many there are. How do you know how to find and build your *True You*?

Easy! You follow your feelings, your sense of attraction to doing something or a feeling of hesitation away from doing something.

I can stop this very moment, close my eyes, and listen to my feelings within. Join me, if you will. Ask yourself the same questions that I ask myself, and then provide your own answer.

Lynn Weiss (LW): Am I happy to be a writer? Yes, as long as I'm interviewing people, writing about people's real lives, and following the wonderful fantasies and creative ideas in my mind that ADD makes possible for me.

Reader: Am I happy to be a _____?

Answer _____

_____

LW: Am I eager to create what I'd like to share with you as a writer? Oh, yes. I love to make language twist and turn and sing to fit the wonderful feelings associated with the meaning of the words in my mind. What an outlet for my ADD sensitivity and rhythm.

Reader: Am I eager to create what I'd like to share with you as a _____?

_____

LW: Does it make me feel honest within myself to write this book and valuable to say, "I am a writer?" Yes, because my goal is to share what I believe in so that others can benefit from my experience.

Reader: Does it make me feel honest within myself to _____ and valuable to say, "I am a _____?" (Be truthful. It's okay to be searching. It took me a lot of time to arrive at my current sense of my *True You*.) _____

_____

_____

LW: What's hard about writing for me? Answer: Sitting still in front of a computer for long hours.

Reader: What's hard for you about pursuing your path?

_____

_____

LW: What's easy about writing for me? It gives me an opportunity to listen to all the interesting things in my head, write about them in story form so I can share them with readers, and then dialogue with the public about our similar experiences. It's the meeting with like-kind that most pleases me.

Reader: What makes it easy for you to follow your path?

_____

_____

My answers to these questions tell me if I'm pursuing a path of value for me. What do your answers tell you?

_____

_____

You notice I don't ask, "How am I judged by the outside world? Is my sense of success based on these judgments?" My answer would be "No." That would not tell me if being a writer is a part of my *True Self*. I may or may not be able to sell what I write. I may or may not reach the target audience with which I desire to dialogue. True, these things would be nice. But whether I'm affirmed from outside of myself doesn't matter as much as the fact that I love the process of writing, touching words that touch feelings that then touch another's feelings and, ultimately, touch their whole being.

In the following paragraphs you will see how to achieve this. You will do a lot of listening to yourself and you will notice what you're attracted to or hesitant about—not hesitant because of fear you'll fail, but the hesitancy brought by trying to do something that you *should* do instead of something you *want* to do.

You have the answers: listen, observe, and practice what calls to you.

If you need money, go get a job that will feed you and your dependents until you can make enough money to transition to your *True You*'s ability to make your living. Or, if need be, continue with your money-making job and spend some time regularly doing what reflects the *True You*. That way you will keep your *True You* alive and healthy. And, that will not only feel good, but will be a very good thing to do.

FINDING YOUR *FIT* IN THE PAST, PRESENT, AND FUTURE

Here's your first assignment.

No one, nor any test, can find your *True You* for you. You can't hire it done. You can't "research it," though you can look, listen, and feel for bits and pieces of it. You may ask for input from others, but first you must look at yourself, including your history, observations, thoughts, and feelings about who you have been and who you are now, who you may wish to become in order to maximize your skills, talents, and wonderful brainstyle, and what you ultimately wish to leave as your legacy for those who follow you.

I'm talking about a process—one that will be under your control. My only job is to give you some ideas to follow. But even these you'll have to assess in order to decide whether what is said *fits* you. Yes, *fits* you. This bold, little three-letter word is the key and King of this whole *True You* phenomenon: *Fit*.

To help you gain clues to finding your *fit*, you will benefit from using some cheat sheets—cheat sheets of characteristics and attributes of various traits, brainstyles, and developmental components that affect the way you are made. Identify with what feels important to you. That will be a clue that guides you toward your *True You*. If you don't identify with one of the characteristics or attributes, it probably tells you that the direction pointed to is not on your path.

Identifying Your Tools

To find the *True You*, we are going to use the Stages of ADD Awareness, the Attributes and the Types of ADD, and the Core Components of Human Nature.

The Stages of ADD Awareness unfold as soon as you recognize that you have an Analogue style of brain construction. It doesn't matter whether you simply identify with the traits or are formally identified or "diagnosed."

Stages of ADD Awareness (Please refer to the Five Stages of ADD, chapter 2, p. 37.)

Stage 1: "Aha, I Have It!"
Stage 2: The Grief Stage
Stage 3: The Family Stage
Stage 4: The Growing Up Stage
Stage 5: Coming of Age

Attributes of ADD (Please refer to chapter 1, p. 11.)

Big Picture Viewer
Patterns and Relationships (way of viewing)
Function (how things function)
Kinesthetic Learner
High Level of Activity (mentally, physically)
Sensitive (in relation to all the senses)
Sensate (an inner knowing)
Rhythmic Timing/Nature (a natural sensing)
Inner Locus of Control (related to sensing)

Types and Forms of ADD

Type I Outwardly Directed: ADD Traits (Example: Belle, chapter 4, p. 124).

- Naturally Active, Spontaneous, High-risk taking, Demonstrative, Quick to change, Reacts to external pressure, Wide mood swings.
- In Linear situations: Easily bored, Short attention span, Dislikes repetition and long-term projects, Expresses temper and frustration, Blames others, Becomes reactive.

Type II Inwardly Directed: ADD without high activity Traits (Example: Jai, chapter 4, p. 129)

- Naturally very empathetic, Slow to change, Visionary/dreamer, Very sensitive, Highly Kinesthetic, Often highly creative, Restless.
- In Linear situation: Tends to blame self, Distractible when bored, Burns out, Tends toward depression, Vacillates, Tries too hard.

Type III Highly Structured ADD Traits (Example: Quentin, chapter 4, p. 134)

- Naturally likes structure, Highly organized, Perfectionistic, Highly focused, Talkative, Dislikes interruptions, Mentally restless, Systematic problem solver, Takes charge in a crisis.
- In Linear situations: Tends to be demanding, Rigid, Judgmental, Obsessively worries, Loses temper, Controlling.

Core Components of Human Nature (CCHN)

Note which of these components are your strengths and which you will need to work on.

A Sense of Trust: Yields security, optimism, consistency, patience, trust, reliability, good listening skills, comfort with intimacy.

A Sense of Self-Awareness: Yields independence, individuality, leadership, ease with sharing, ability to set goals and make decisions.

A Sense of Competence: Yields expressiveness, curiosity, willingness to try new things, ability to recoup from mistakes and failures, perspective on a job, self-motivation, ability to ask questions, creativity.

A Sense of Powerfulness: Yields ability to be responsible, state what one wants, be assertive not aggressive, say "no," win or lose, use good judgment, follow through on commitments, be an honest effective manager, implement goals, ideas, and dreams, defend self and others appropriately.

A Sense of Self-Control: The ability to maintain control of one's behavior based on impulse control, purposeful letting go of control, and one's value system.

Sense of Self-Control—Impulsivity: Yields reliability, predictability, good judgment, responsibility for actions, self-monitoring, and balance.

Sense of Self-Control—Letting Go (of control on purpose): Yields empathy, playfulness, high morale with coworkers, sets work priorities that are realistic, avoids burnout, and accepts help when needed.

A Sense of Self-Control—Value System: Value system has been thought through in adult life, is firm but relative, has eliminated *shoulds* from actions, acts out of belief rather than fear or to please another, and is comfortable with values different from own.

Exploring Your True *Fit*

Now that you've completed a review of your cheat sheets, what I ask you to do is to go back through this list of categories and again consider the items under each heading that seem to fit you. Don't judge yourself. The intent is to guide you to assets that will help you and difficulties that you will benefit from working on or situations to avoid.

You will see how different dimensions affect the composite that makes you up. What a wonderful mix you are. You'll find areas in which you have strength and other areas where you need to pump up your emotional, cognitive, or social muscle. That's fine— because no one has the whole package all put together. And, besides, it will keep you busy in your spare time.

Remembering and Dreaming

Write a sentence, a paragraph or two, or a page of whatever comes to your mind when the words *True You* are mentioned. There are no rules about this. Write to yourself. No one else needs to see what you've written . . . or they can if you wish. Forget about grammar. And make it as short or long as you wish.

Oh yes, and if writing is absolutely not your thing, draw a picture, a schematic or use modeling clay or any material that captures the sense of *You*. You may dance a dance or play an instrument or do something athletically physical.

You will not be able to keep *You* out of what you do. And there are no limits to the form of the expression. In fact, later on in this chapter, you will find a story that will show you just how "out of the box" a *True You* set of attributes can manifest.

It's even okay to jump ahead if you're stumped on your own, but first rely on yourself to become aware of what comes to you. You see, by just reading these words, your psyche will begin to stimulate that part of you that has been wanting you to pay attention your entire life. Please don't cheat yourself.

Here are a few questions to stimulate your remembering and dreaming. Be sure that you have paper and pencil/pen nearby to make notes or draw pictures or "whatever." Remember to listen and feel what comes to your attention.

Do you remember a time when you lay on the ground looking straight up at the clouds and daydreamed about what you might do as an adult?

Do you recall overhearing your parents, a counselor, or others say what they thought you'd be good doing when you grow up?

Do you remember watching a TV show or reading a book about a character who was playing a role that made you want to be just like that?

As you consider any of these questions, jot down what your reactions are. You don't need to respond to all of them, only the ones that interest you. Or if one makes you think of something else, then capture the thoughts it stimulates.

Remember, this is for you. You're not taking a test as if you're in school.

Consider Your History and Thinking

When did you grow up? What years? When were you a teen, a young adult? Eight years old? What was going on in the culture at the time? War, social expansion, bankruptcies, inflation, creativity (as in the American 1960s,) etc.

I recall being a teen during the pre–Women's Lib time. My dad had suffered from not having a "profession." So he insisted that I had to get one. His insistence stemmed from a combination of having been a young man during the Great Depression (a very financially scary time), having a wife (my mother) with a minimal education that left her unmarketable, and my being an only child who was a creative dreamer in a society with a father who believed that such people couldn't make a living using those skills.

I recall being very confused, and it took me years to get some of the repercussions straight about who I am and what I really want to do. Finally, I gave myself permission to do what I wanted. Luckily for me, I was drawn into the Anti-Poverty and Community Mental Health Programs of the 1960s followed by Head Start for preschool children's education that helped bring equity to children's education in the United States. Each of these programs fit my skills, talents, and interests in the arena of cultural anthropology, social relationships, and community organization.

As my professional evolution unfolds many years later, I'm finding a very different market that will require different skill sets than those that are a natural part of my *True Self*—technology and administrative management being two. This requires me to partner with others who have a more Linear orientation to balance my skills and interests in order to spread the word about ADD as a Diversity Issue. I need to use my creativity to find new ways to bring support and assistance to Analogue processors in a manner that is neither costly nor pathologizing of people with a perfectly wonderful style of brain construction.

So you see, it is imperative to consider the culture and communities in which you were raised and in which you are currently living. As I mentioned earlier in the book, small towns often make better, easier locales for ADD people to live and make a living naturally at less loss to their *True Self*. There tend to be more kinesthetic, hands-on opportunities to make a living. This could suit you just fine.

Exploring Your True Timing: Is It Time?

By now, you may have a preferred way in which to capture your exploration of your *True Self*. Let's look at your readiness to figure out your current *True You*.

When you begin to feel restless or disappointed with what you are currently doing, you may begin to consider other options. This could be good. It may be that the question will create restlessness in you. And this stands for a sign that can awaken your *True You* energy. You'll need to consider your current situation. Ask yourself the following questions:

Are you at a place in life that has a natural transition associated with it?

For example, are you leaving school for the workplace, not as a part-time job to keep you in school, but as a way of asserting your independence and getting on with your life?

Or have you just retired from a major career? Perhaps you aren't ready to stop working and feel a little or a lot excited about pursuing a heart-felt interest?

Has your whole life turned upside down because your spouse walked out on you and your head is swimming as you wonder who you are and how you'll financially survive?

In these situations, it may or may not be the right time to pursue your *True Self*. On the one hand, it might not be the right time to jump into *True You* work. On the other hand, it may be exactly the right time to go for broke with a sort of "why not?" attitude.

Let's say you are fed up with school or getting close to flunking out. You must first deal with your feelings of anger or loss or feelings of being a failure before you jump into another goal-oriented endeavor. This is totally different from dropping out of school temporarily, especially with a fixed time limit, so you can figure out the direction that you want to go in school toward your degree. In the latter situation, you purposely withdraw so that you can reenter free and clear when you are ready. That way you are in control of your situation.

Meanwhile, you will be doing two things: making a living and exploring the direction that you want to take to make the best use of your talents and interests on your way to getting a credential or degree that you think will *fit* the person you want to become.

Another scenario may appear because you get a raise at your current job and suddenly find that you don't like the new job, but instead, preferred the work that you had been doing. For example, teachers who love to teach and are promoted to be administrators face this all the time. Hands-on professionals who are suddenly elevated to management may suffer the same loss of love for their work.

Timing and Rhythm Come Into Play

Timing and rhythm are crucial to your changes. Be sure to check with yourself to see what your timing system desires and needs. One of the natural attributes of ADD is our propensity to follow our own unique timing and move with the flow of speed that most pleases us. If you have a primarily ADD brainstyle, speed may be your best friend, letting you know that your restlessness is trying to tell you something about your situation. Have you been sitting at a desk too long?

Please acknowledge the possibility to your inner sensory system that maybe it is time to move on, because you have acknowledged previously that you are due for a move every three or four years or are plain bored with what you're doing.

Oh, and by the way, if someone tells you that you shouldn't move that often, tell them "thank you" for their concern and go ahead and move. To be sure, you must consider why you've changed jobs. But as long as you are paying your bills; considering others in your family; not changing because you're involved with drugs, alcohol, or behavior that is addictive or illegal in any way; or because you're picking fights with authority figures and the like—then trust yourself. This does mean you must be honest with yourself and live a psychologically responsible life.

I've known several Type I and Type II ADD people who have spent their entire lives working through temp agencies. (Agencies that send people into businesses to work on a specific job or when a full-time employee has to take a temporary leave.) In several of these instances, the individuals have had side passions such as music, or the love of spending time in the outdoors, or had a hobby that they want to pursue. The temporary work is consistent and pays the bills and they don't need to rely on trying to make a living by demanding that someone else bring in the steady income.

Interestingly, some people stay in the same job their entire career because of a need or desire to have the security of a steady paycheck. They may not love their career, but their need for security trumps their desire to do something they would savor. When the time comes that they are able to retire, they may find a sweet time of being able to play with the true desire of their heart. On the other hand, maybe they actually have been quite content with what they had been doing all those years.

Timing and rhythm are crucial. Be sure to check with yourself to see what your timing system desires and needs.

What Can You Not "Not Do?"

Glance back over the years prior to now. Even as a kid, did you have a hobby, a preferred recreational outlet, a favorite, often repeated vacation experience or a field of learning that you pursued year after year?

CJ always played soccer, then became a referee. And no matter what he did for work, where he lived, or what stage in life he found himself, he gravitated to the soccer fields where he felt his very best. His *True Self* was and is related to soccer.

Judy traveled with her family as a child and could hardly wait for the next vacation time to arrive so they would head out for new and exotic places. She eventually earned her college degree in a foreign language, became a foreign-student director, and met people from all over the world. Every vacation meant travel somewhere to spend time with the families and friends of her students as well as embracing the local culture in all of its glory.

At one point, she became a Peace Corps volunteer and spent two additional years teaching ESL (English as a Second Language) in the geographic area of her original assignment in Eastern Europe. After a year in the United States, she was off to buy property in South America and became an expatriate for eight years. Having returned to the States to help out with family needs, she is already planning her next travels when she finds time to get away.

Judy is extremely content being who she is and living the way she has lived all these years. She has absolutely no interest in changing her *True You* vision. Meanwhile, she keeps up with international issues through friends, local programs, and television movies and documentaries from all around the world.

This woman's *True Self* is that of a perennial traveler. And, the most interesting thing is that she does it on extremely little money and always has. She simply *fits* the rhythm and movement of a traveler who makes friends all over the world.

Different Journeys for Different Folks

Again I ask you to take time with yourself—without input from others at this point—to consider that probably no two of us are the same. Needless to say, neither will be our journeys to find our *True Selves*. So you're on your own in discovering your *True Self*, though not without support.

The next section will set you to thinking, writing, and trying things out. So settle yourself into a space and time that will allow you and your inner self to have a good dialogue with your thinking, feeling, and listening self. Follow up by turning some of what you gain in this way into a mini real-life adventure, experiment, or trial.

What Do You Think/Feel Your Raw Material Is?

Are you mostly an Analogue processing person? _____
Are you mostly a Linear processing person? _____
Are you a Bridge person (part Analogue/part Linear)? _____

When it comes to feeling and thinking about the *True You*, you must look at how the different types of processing guide you. For example, if you have Linear attributes, such as Bridge People do, you will tend to think strategically and cognitively about these questions in relation to yourself, at least part of the time. Making a list of why you think the way you do may serve you. You could look at the traits involved and assess your strengths and weakness in these areas. Planning may become your best friend. You may ask others to evaluate you. Being excited about what you achieve is likely.

If, however you are primarily an Analogue processing person, you'll tend to *feel* your way through what feels right and what doesn't. You'll likely be hard put to come up with reasons why you choose to follow the path you believe you want to follow. You also may be almost totally unwilling to think about not doing what touches your heart. Being passionate about what you want to do is not an unusual response.

Parameters of Your Path

Born to be Free! Ah, I hear the music playing. And, indeed, some of us were born to move toward our *True Selves* as if it were coded in our DNA.

Born to Your *True You* Path. Do you have the feeling of having been born to a particular vocation, career, or life-long interest? Nothing else ever showed up that caught your attention—in fact, nothing else seemed to be able to get through to your conscious awareness as a suitable interest to pursue. You probably had no doubts about a choice that made itself for you.

Do you recall having had an interest in what you wanted to do when you grew up, but then became aware of other directions you felt you might like? Exploration may have wooed you to expand your initial blueprint of interest. In time you may have found yourself quite content to stay with your secondary or tertiary interest. Actually it's possible that your *True Self* has multiple facets. No one said you had to stay with a monolithic model.

So many, many things interested you. You'd try one thing for a while and then switch to something else, and so on—and your family and teachers supported your choices. Occasionally you may have found yourself going back to an earlier interest. Each time you found yourself engaged in an interest, you felt fully immersed and recall thinking that perhaps "This is it."

Very likely you have a mixture of traits that may or may not combine into one activity. Rather you just may be "Living the Process of your United _True You_, not living one vision of a _True Self_."

Now you see that you have some expanded ways to look at your _True Self_. No one way is the one right way to go about being Yourself. Enjoy the journey and consider whether you are a "One Point" Person, a "Multiple Point" Person, or a "United Process" Person.

The best news is that you will know when you arrive at your pattern. Don't limit the way it comes about or looks as a finished product. Let yourself become what you are naturally and then describe what it is about rather than saying what you need to be and then being saddened when you are not the way you thought you _ought_ to be.

DEALING WITH YOUR _TRUE YOU_

Zero to Sixty in How Long?

Timing is a fascinating aspect of trying to discover where you are going. We don't all poke our little heads up out of the garden soil at the same time and grow at the same pace. We don't all reach our maturity at the same time. That is how nature works. And we have to learn to deal with it.

In the beginning, you may have no interest in such an exercise as finding a _True You_. So you go for a walk around the park. Or you may choose to take off like a sprinter determined to finish first in search of your *True Self*.

Then again, you may be drawn to marathon running where you're in the race for the long haul. Steadiness and rhythm are your best friends as you pace yourself and find that runner's high to cruise in for as long as you like where it doesn't even seem that you are running.

Finally, there is the relay race with each part of the foursome playing a special role. Each position requires runners to have specific skills. Each is important in its own way. So, you, too, may start slowly and then pick up speed as you proceed as if there are different aspects of yourself that are a part of your run.

Or in contrast, you may start quickly, like the proverbial canon shot until the time comes to cruise in order to collect your thoughts. Many people are happy to get their security protected before going for their merry-go-round ring. Others would prefer not to mix their emotional attachments with money-making security. Give yourself the opportunity to let your *True Self* deal in its own way.

Let Your Self Unfold In Its Own Time

You may give yourself the benefit of knowing your *True You* even if you don't focus on it right away. It may not be your first issue of importance. Take for example someone who lived with serious poverty as a child and never again wants to have to feel badly about money, and so blocks out everything else until security is a sure thing. Then the *True You* search can be taken up.

In Addition to My *True Self*, I Want . . .

Place a number from 1 to 5 next to each of the following goals that may be associated with your adult life. 1 equals not very important. 5 means very important.

money _____   popularity _____
status _____   fame _____
freedom of choice _____   security _____
self-employment _____   attention _____
ambition _____   play _____
creative _____   laid-back _____
self-support _____   other _____

Where Else Might Signs of Your *True Self* Be Hiding?

Self-study, much of which you'll bump into throughout this book and other self-help, growth, and motivational goals books, may take top priority. Or you may want to read biographies, autobiographies, and memoirs. Don't forget to observe public entertainment, in person, on TV and radio, and through local lectures. Get to see what people are doing with their lives. Look around you in new environments and see what people do with their time.

Finally, there are specialty magazines that often highlight biographical material of participants noted in their articles. A library or bookstore full of magazines may be a good resource. College continuing education programs, and local parks and recreation centers serve up hundreds of opportunities to see what the world is made of.

All you have to do is watch with the following question in your mind: Does this interest me? Do I feel drawn to this? Do I feel a twinge of excitement or interest in what is happening here? Would I like to entertain the idea of being a part of this sort of activity? You don't have to like the whole activity. There may be a small part of it you are drawn to.

Pay attention to how you feel. Happy, sad, bored, excited, or curious about trying it.

Ferreting Out the Simple Things

Finally, do not overlook the simple things in life. One workshop I did involved mothers and daughters. When one teen was asked what she liked to do, both she and her mother verbalized a family belief: "Nothing."

It took a little querying to elicit one of the most basic answers I have ever heard.

> **Lynn Weiss (LW) to Mother** after discovering that the girl had no stated hobbies, or activities: What does your daughter do when she gets home from school each day?
>
> **Mother**: Nothing
>
> **LW to Mother**: Does she walk through the front door?
>
> **Mother**: Yes.
>
> **LW to Mother**: Just bear with me for a minute, okay? Then what does she do?
>
> **Mother**: She goes in the kitchen and gets a snack.
>
> **LW to Mother**: Then?
>
> **Mother**: She goes upstairs to her room and I don't see her until dinnertime.

I looked at the daughter and mother as I asked the next question.

> **LW to Mother and Daughter**: And in [her] your room, what do you do?
>
> **Daughter**: I talk on the phone to my friends.
>
> **LW to Daughter**: What do you find to talk about for all that time?

The Mother jumped in with the answer: "She has a lot of friends who call her with their problems and she really helps them. She's been doing it for several years now."

With that answer I saw a smile of pride and pleasure come to the daughter's lips. Wow, the teen turned out to be a helper-counselor type of person.

LW to Daughter: You must be a really good listener . . . and must give good advice since your friends keep wanting to talk with you. Ever thought of becoming a counselor one day?

Daughter: Oh, I'd love that.

LW to Mother and Daughter: Well, why don't you all investigate what it takes to be a mental health aide or a counselor. You look like that might open some doors to who you are growing up to be: your *True You*. If, after getting into it, you start losing interest or find something else that intrigues you, you won't have lost anything because you'll know that much more about yourself. And the skills that you learn on the way you will probably use in ways you never dreamed.

Barricades and Detours

Take a few moments to check and see whether some old worries, *shoulds* or distractions of your making, are coming into play. Don't be surprised if moving closer to finding the *True You* stirs up some concerns and makes you feel poorly emotionally or even physically.

You need not pay attention to mild ups and downs of emotions. That's normal whenever we work toward creating change. But if your attention is called to an old wounding or you sense yourself being drawn in an emotional direction that you've visited before and you know it is not a good place for you to visit, then stop working your program temporarily and return to the healing ways that stabilized you previously.

Check in with a counselor if necessary. Counselors all know that change stirs the pot. You will learn this, too. You won't be starting over with your healing. Rather, you'll find that your wounded part, with help, will quickly remember the healing that occurred previously and will be delighted to jump-start recovery for your benefit.

Check outside pressures: Chronic Stress Response, life issues including finances, jobs, relationships (new and old), family issues and disease, adding a child to the family, discovering that a child is handicapped, dealing with aging parents, or needing to respond to emergencies with family or friends. Those are but a few.

With these, remember that you can do everything, just not at the same time. Such interruptions do not mean that you can never return to your work/life that you desire, but it may mean putting things on hold for a while. Even stress situations often have a time during their course when you can breathe and consider what you've been experiencing.

Maybe you'd like to do some dreaming. Maybe your current experience is adding fodder for the future evolution of your *True You*. If you need to let go of your dream for a while, have a special place to put it for the time being. But don't fully let go of the dream. Give yourself hope by making a symbol or verse that captures your soaring self. Then put the symbol (picture, item, journal) on display where you can readily walk past it periodically. From time to time, breathe in and say, "thank you" to your symbol for being there to provide you with hope. You've done well by yourself and you'll continue to do well.

Everything truly comes to an end. It just seems as if it won't when we're caught in a whirlpool of emotion. Roadblocks take time to clear, but eventually they open up. Consider ways to use your time in your own best interest and for the good of all while you're looking for opportunities to pursue your dream actively.

The Critic

Watch out for the Inner Critic, a voice in your head with which you weren't born but that has been heard repeatedly as if recorded and replayed ad infinitum. Why not use this as a good time to silence it through your Sense of Powerfulness to get your own needs met, as you set limits on what you do not want in your territory?

Begin by thinking about when you first heard The Critic. Were you a kid, teen, young adult, or older person?

Next think about what you had been doing right before The Critic arrived.

_____

_____

Recall how you felt right before The Critic arrived.

_____

_____

How did you feel after The Critic had arrived?

_____

_____

Do you know what The Critic wants?

_____

_____

What is the job that The Critic is trying to accomplish?

_____

_____

How else can that job be accomplished now?

_____

_____

You will find that you may have outgrown that original voice of The Critic. But as with a persistent irritant of any kind, your mind got used to it and every time you listened to it, you inadvertently reinforced it. You can kindly ask it to go away. Be sure to tell it "thank you" for trying to work on your behalf. Then say that you've grown older now and, having developed good judgment, you will take over the job it has done for so long.

If The Critic is persistent and unwilling to leave, you can also go to an isolated place and yell at it. After thanking it for having taken care of you for so very long, sternly tell it that you are going to take over the job now. Any time after that when it pops back into your consciousness, firmly say something like, "Out of here!" You may have to repeat that for a period of time, but you have a very good chance of extinguishing it.

Finally, hypnosis can finish the job if your Critic is particularly stubborn. Please, don't feel down on yourself because it only means that you have a lot of wonderful energy that will become available to apply in your best interest once the energy of The Critic is redirected.

We've already taken a look at sociocultural values that we learned at an early age. Sometimes these values house a Critic because we learned that doing a particular thing or being a particular way is wrong.

I recall when I was in my twenties and I was just beginning to practice counseling in Southern California. One beautiful October day, I finished a school consultation in the early afternoon and thought how wonderful it would be to drive north on the Pacific Coast Highway in my awesome first new car bought with my first "real" earnings: a yellow Karmann Ghia Convertible. (Three years of monthly payments @ $78.00/month.)

I hadn't gone more than two blocks in that direction when suddenly I was struck by a tightness in my stomach and a guilty feeling the size of a house pressing against my heart. I pulled over and thought about what was happening. What I discovered still amazes me.

First of all, I saw that I'd imagined a small figure about three inches tall standing on my right shoulder, pointing a finger at me, scolding me for even thinking of taking off for the beach on a Thursday afternoon.

"What?" I exclaimed out loud. "Where did you come from?"

In my mind, the little guy looked like the McDonald's "Hamburglar" in his big black hat and black coat. That was my first visual meeting with my Critic.

As I thought about what was happening I realized the problem. It was a weekday afternoon and I held a belief that I must work from 8 a.m. Monday morning until 6 p.m. Friday afternoon. Only then could I take time off and play. This, of course came from years of being in school as a child and young adult.

On this particular day, I had planned to write up my clinical notes. But they weren't due until the next morning and I could easily write in the evening after the beautiful, warm, fall sun began to move below the horizon. I thought, "Why not trade the afternoon time for the evening time?"

The final clincher was that I knew what a highly responsible person I was and if I decided to make this time shift, there would be no question that I would do what I planned by finishing the reports in the evening. So, I turned the motor back on, said "Good-bye" to the little man, and drove away momentarily free of my critic.

A few minutes later he reappeared, again pointing his finger at my head. I said, "Thank you for teaching me to be responsible, but now you can go on away. I've taken over your job." I think he'd come back because I'd forgotten to say, "Thank you" earlier when I first drove off.

I had almost reached the Santa Monica beach when he momentarily reappeared. Laughing, I nodded my head in his direction and said, firmly, but with a chuckle, "Out of here!" That was the last time I ever saw Mr. Hamburglar.

Mr. Critic has lots of helper critics in this world. You'll need to watch out for them and question whether you want to believe in what they have to say or not.

Try going to a writers' group. There you'll find more would-be experts per square inch than ants in an ant hill. You will need to be prepared to consider how you want to handle your work as a writer. You can submit your work for scrutiny if you truly want a variety of input. Or, perhaps you simply want to share because you are very pleased that you've achieved your own personal goal in your writing.

What's being measured is not a value or perfection of the writing, but the listener's pleasure with the writing. It's the listener who likes the way in which the writing is expressed. The major issue is that brainstyles strongly impact the preference of listener and viewer. Linear people often tend to prefer more structured, dense, complicated literature with lots of details like names of people and places. Analogue readers may prefer a sensory experience that flows and builds pictures and stories for your minds to visualize. Neither type is better than the other—they are simply diverse writing styles—though there is a cultural tendency to think that the Linear approach is better, smarter, more complex and sophisticated and, therefore, more worthy of winning competitions and being the *right* way.

Here's the Judge

You have one more ally, should you wish to call upon your Inner Judge. If you do, set yourself up as the judge and have a parole hearing.

Present the facts about yourself. Remember, if you're talking to a judge, you have to take an oath to tell the truth, the whole truth, and nothing but the truth.

Check, "I will" _____.

List the reasons why you are ready to take responsibility for your own needs, wants, and desires. Muster your courage to say what others may not understand, but that you know within yourself you'd really like to own, in the sense of belonging to you.

Make a list of the points that you want to present to your Inner Judge. Next, take a deep breath and proceed to take the step of trusting yourself. And finally, hear the judge bellow, "You're Freed!"

Off you go to live your life, not as a life that someone or something else scripted for you. You're in charge and free!

If you're a sensitive, Analogue person, be clear that it is up to you to self-protect if you need and want to. Choose the settings in which you put your heart on the line and expose your sensitivity to criticism. First and foremost, you must like and approve of your own work regardless of what others think. That will add to your growing your *True You*.

GROWING THE *TRUE YOU*

Signs of Wrong and Right Paths

You've experimented. You've learned to clear the path to your *True You*, and now you're ready to Grow It.

Nothing is black or white in the flow of life. Certainly finding the *True You* isn't. Neither is the flow of the five stages of the Core Components of Human Nature that feed the manifestation of your *True You*.

Finding the *True You* is a truly Analogue process that flows, stops, starts, slows down, turns around, and dances to its own tune. So you're not out anything if the path you're treading is a bit erratic, twisting and turning, and causes a flat tire here and there.

Always leave room for restarting and stopping as needed. Learning what doesn't work is as important as having early success that may often change and that you have no experience at fixing, changing, and building anew.

Above all, do not hold on too tight. It would seem that the tighter you hold onto what is from the past or in the now, the more you'll be subjected to stress in order to dislodge you from your comfort zone. It's rather like standing up against a wave at the ocean that will knock you over on your backside if you insist on trying to stand up against it. Rather you may have learned to dive through the wave and roll backward with the flow of its movement while experiencing the vibrant energy of the water.

As you are pursuing your *True Self*, watch out for signs that you're on the Wrong Path doing something you don't really want to do. Several common signs include: strong emotional responses and negative or stressful feelings, feelings of depression, anxiety, and hesitant feelings, or you may repeatedly run into obstacles, problems, objections, and the like.

Such signs may mean you're on the Wrong Path, but they also may indicate a problem with timing. When you begin to feel poorly or encounter obstacles, gently explore within yourself whether you're trying to rush things, do too much too fast, not prepare your foundation properly, or balance the discovery of the *True You* within the context of other aspects of yourself and your life. You may have an unconscious block that is restricting the success of your manifesting your *True You*. It's also possible that the world is not ready yet for what you have to offer.

Maybe you're trying to recapture a part of your past that was quite nice, but it is, in fact, past. Sometimes we are drawn to what had felt so good and, since we don't know what will come, it can be a lot more comfortable reaching back for the known rather than forward to the unknown.

Give yourself some leeway. Back off for a while and see what happens. Look for related ways to be yourself. Maybe it is only a matter of the time.

Watch out for signs that you're on the Right Path doing something that fits the *True You*. Thinly dissect what you're doing so you can analyze what is working for you. You may be able to apply it to the negative responses that cross your path above.

Signs of being on a Right Path include: feeling happy, enthusiastic, joyful, contented, loving, appreciative, and energetic. Keep your eyes open for good news.

What I Wish I Had Done . . .

Not an unknown statement from the mouths of so many. And it's not just elders who realize time may be running out as they recognize that there were things they didn't do that they really wanted to do. You are not alone. So, let's tackle this issue head on.

Try Writing:

If only I had, as an adult, followed through on my childhood dreams, finished school, did what I wanted to do that I was told wasn't sensible, saved money or _____ _____ so I could _____ _____

The Unfinished business that I wish I'd finished was/is

_____
_____

Why not finish it now? _____

_____

Try again. Why not? _____

_____

You might be having a tough time answering this question. If so, your job now is to work with a counselor, teacher, mentor, or your own self to find the rough spot(s) that you're hung up on. When you do, come back here and write in what you found.

_____
_____

Then get back on the path and head to the *True You* that you're meant to reach.

Self-Quiz Time

What were you born to do? (You might want to watch the movie *Secretariat* [the horse that won the triple crown though he wasn't even supposed to be a winner of anything]. He ended up just being himself in his own way. The judges and critics didn't think he had it in him. But, the truth was that Secretariat was born to run.)

What about You? What were you born to do?

_____

_____

_____

Differentiate between what you're good at from what you like/love to do. Make a list.

Like to Do	Love to Do

Circle Your Preferences: Where or what would you prefer to be associated with in order to carry out the role of your *True You*. Would you rather be:

Stationary or Active
Indoors or Outdoors
Front Stage or Back Stage
A Loner or A Groupie
A Feelings Person or A Thinking Person
Hands-on Doer or Planner and Thinker How to Do
Linear Strategist or Analogue Strategist
What makes you:
Comfortable _____
Uncomfortable _____

Special interest(s) worth saving for and skipping dessert:

_____

_____

TWO TYPES OF GROWTH EXPERIENCES

I'd like to finish this section by introducing two people, HJ and Nadine, who touched me in very different ways and represent diverse attempts to find their *True Selves*. Each had the sense of something within them that they wanted to reach, but didn't have the words or guidance to know what it was.

Unlike physical capabilities that can become apparent early on in gym class and peewee sports programs, many of the attributes that represent the creative, special, heart-enriching art of ourselves don't show themselves so easily. Oh, sure, there are other talents that show readily in classes, groups, competitions, and activities. But when the talent, interest, and special desires are less tangible, then it's not very easy to identify them.

Success on the Way: HJ

At thirty-four, HJ sought counseling. Old enough to be confused, but smart enough to ask for help, it turns out this was a best-steps scenario for him to take.

He is good looking, fit, employed, addiction-free, and behaviorally sound. He looks good on the surface. But inside, he reported he felt restless, not just because he is ADD, but because . . . well, he didn't quite know why, but he sensed that he wanted more out of life. Corny? A bit, perhaps. But, you see, HJ has many skills and interests and enough mental health to be happy, but when he realized that his restlessness wasn't just because of being ADD, he thought better of letting it remain as an impediment in his life.

When he found a psychologist who knew a lot about ADD as well as being a well-rounded clinician, he followed his intuition and booked time. The major area that he focused on was his career, hopes, expectations, and what might be getting in the way for him.

As is often helpful, they looked at the impact of HJ's early years. Though his mother died at his birth, that didn't seem to be a pivotal problem, and his father took responsibility to raise his son. But HJ spent much time with his paternal grandfather who was a carpenter, always building something with HJ right by his side. Not only did their relationship fit HJ's core skill base, but it was nurturing, so his emotional needs also were met.

HJ was rather shy, but always had a group of boys who he hung with who were, by his description, "Geeks." They were very loyal to one another and enjoyed the same activities including playing in a band and designing video games.

A wounding occurred when, with no warning, his father moved the family (now including a step mom) out of state, which mainly disrupted HJ's social network and caused him havoc in high school. He found himself way behind the other students in his new school and spent a year and a half catching up. He described himself as someone who didn't do homework but "soaked up" the school material.

The destabilization in those early and mid-teen years set HJ up for a chaotic entry into his young adult world. He and his father disagreed about where he was to start college and what he'd major in. Turns out he was intuitively drawn to a track that was important to his core self. He really liked video game designing as well as hands-on software engineering.

Unfortunately, HJ lost touch with an orderly, supportive structure as he pressed to become his own person on a road to his *True Self*. Without the guidance and support of an adult, he washed up on shore without the credentials and certifications he needed to get employed at what he loved—video-game design.

Back and forth without guidance that supported what he loved at his core, HJ ended up in a corporate job that was devoid of attention to his artistic and design interests. He did like the hands-on technical work of engineering, however. Luckily for him, this all came to a head when he was asked to go into management, which he didn't want to do. As an engineer, he said, "I am awesome. I can fix anything and create endlessly. Just don't ask me to create daily status reports!" That says it all.

It was this struggle—between hands-on work with which he felt comfortable and administration that didn't much fit his brainstyle and experience—that drove HJ into psychotherapy where he gained the understanding and direction he needed to realize the inner forces driving him. What a gift!

He discovered something was incongruent inside his psyche. Something was missing. He felt somewhat of a phony at work, not because he wasn't capable of doing his job, but because he had to keep hidden a part of who he was, that is, his ADD brainstyle characteristics. It is likely that he was afraid that if people really knew him, they would judge and criticize him the way his family did as he was growing up. To survive, HJ internalized much of this parental judgment with one result being that his own Inner Critic had grown to be very powerful, out of control, and more harmful than helpful.

He's had to learn to regulate his Inner Critic so that it could support his multifaceted development. He began doing this. As a result he's become more psychologically flexible and courageous, thus becoming willing to experiment with new behaviors. He began to catch up with accommodations he was intuitively learning to use to balance his ADD brainstyle so that he could make choices that, at first, didn't seem possible.

One of HJ's responses has been to take art classes and also return to refurbishing his skills so he can work on his own video-game development ideas. He can now look into the mirror reflecting his *True Self* and see the bigger picture of who he really is.

As his therapist put it, "I can guess HJ's psyche was stagnant for many years and now. Perhaps with a little encouraging therapy fertilizer and weed pulling it is naturally growing and flowering."

And so, HJ is on the way with a boost from therapy to integrate his wonderful ADD brainstyle into a life lived in a Linear culture. When I last heard from him, he was again being presented with promotion opportunities at the corporation where he works. This time, he's not experiencing angst. Instead, he is considering the more integrated parts of himself as partners on a journey where he can be and do what he feels is the right thing for him at this time, without abandoning and ignoring other parts of himself that he wishes to continue to cultivate in time. Indeed, Success is on the Way.

Life for HJ may continue on a two-fold path or he may decide further down the road to shift from his current path to another one. Either way, he can make such a decision with solid experience behind him, when he's gotten all he wants out of one path's journey. He may then find that it's time for a shift.

Some of us call it "burn out." That's really not a bad thing. Rather it may simply mean that we've gone as far as our psyches wish, as far as there are lively adventures and new things to learn. When the scenery becomes boring, it may be time to move.

Age can make a difference, and other factors in life, such as wanting to spend more time with our family, may call to us. Perhaps the empty nest opens doorways to our freedom of motion. We can have it all, just not all at the same time.

The *True You* needs to keep the flexibility of youth alive with the stability of growing mature. Together there is opportunity to live fully if we look to the future, respect the past, and live in the present.

Sometimes Things Don't Work Out So Well: Nadine

Nadine at age sixty-plus has had an uphill life. Yes, ADD is her brainstyle. But each of us is made up of many aspects, any of which can go awry. The whole premise of the *True You* is that by finding your right *fit* and then channeling that into doing something with your life that you love, you'll have a chance to be pleased with yourself and find more happiness than not. But, the right *fit* may be out of reach if other parts of us intrude in the fulfillment.

With a brainstyle that was little recognized in her youth—and when it did surface, it was as a "condition" different from the mainstream culture, including the educational system that was based on a Linear model of learning—Nadine failed to be given the education that would help her utilize her intelligence. The result, as you will see, was wounding of a common variety. Wound her it did, primarily by creating low self-confidence, a fear of failure, and a tendency to overanalyze situations and tasks, in addition to not learning ways to accommodate her brainstyle in specific situations. Each wounding left her more fragmented, keeping her from becoming a stable, well-rounded adult.

These wounds didn't need to be there if—and it is a big "if"—she had received understanding and help about the relationship between the Linear and the Analogue styles of thinking and ordering of the world around her. If she had experienced primary nurturing as a child that would have promoted healthy emotional growth to adulthood, and if her biochemistry had allowed her to remain somewhat balanced emotionally, she may have been able to find a pathway to follow that could lead her to a deserved goal of her heart instead of slamming her into culverts at the side of the road.

But these "ifs" didn't happen. Instead she bent from the stress of not knowing how to straighten out her life and ended up moving around in circles that kept repeating the damage.

When we look at her adult work life, you will see how she could not have found her way to her *True You* because those trying to help her did not know what to do either. As a result, she attempted to analyze her own way through her inability to find how to live, earn money, and discover what she liked—all the time becoming more hopeful on one hand and more despairing on the other.

After consulting with a doctor in an attempt to get a diagnosis of ADD in the hopes of finding some community-support services, she was told, "You can't possibly be ADD because you have a college degree." This comment, heard by many adults with an Analogue brainstyle is, of course, totally irrelevant to the identification of ADD. Sadly she did not have the benefit of the supposed college degree because, in reality, it was a two-year college degree that took her six years to accomplish and had no continuity to lead her to a work goal or a *True You* connection for herself.

Another social-service worker called her "odd and eccentric." As it turned out, that was all right with her because her mind translated that into "Creative, and one who sees outside the box." This could have been a clue for Nadine that—had she known to follow it—could have led her to her *True You*.

It was at this point that she was within three months of running out of cash at age sixty, while longing to coach children with ADD. Without a structured path to finding an income that would care for her basic needs, Nadine could not gather her resources together to reach this goal—one that actually may have *fit* her just fine. She simply didn't have the network and guidance behind her from which to draw.

Nadine did not fully grasp the importance of her creative desire and attraction that were trying to lead her to her *True You*. The problem is that her creativity is unstructured and mentally jumps around from one goal to another. When she heard about a job caring for elders, she was so excited that she was sure the job was meant for her. Again it might have *fit* her if she could be stable enough to interview successfully and remain balanced while working at something that was a potential good *fit*. But those outcomes were never tested because she was not called to interview for it. "How demoralizing," she reported.

Nadine's inner child consistently showed signs of wanting to do nurturing work. At one time she'd be drawn to children, the next time to elders, another time to kittens, and so on. Each encounter and dream brought great joy to her. Her own inner needs for the building of her personal need for nurturance and *trust*—a Core Component feature (chapter 2, p. 43)—could have been matched to a job as a caregiver and likely would have fulfilled her true need, if not desire. But the desire to be a nurturer was not recognized to be a consistent thread in her job search.

It wasn't long after being turned down for the elder-caregiving job that she was diagnosed with bipolar disorder and put on medication. Finally, she received help for another difficulty that had laid hidden, wreaking havoc for decades. The medication helped enough that she was able to stay on a job for nearly a year with clients whom she described as "impaired and some who were very hard to deal with." In addition, she said, "I'm having problems with my mean, nasty coworker." So she quit her job and is going for more tests because she sleeps a lot and is tired all the time.

In the same breath, Nadine talked of caring for a young mother cat and four-week-old kittens. "Such joy," she exclaimed.

Most of what has happened to Nadine, who once said her goal was to gravitate toward people in organizations who were aware of Deep Thinkers, is not due to her ADD style of brain construction. Instead, she has a whole lifetime of social, physical, educational, and emotional difficulties that, no doubt, left her with fragmented systems of living and growing that could not take advantage of her ADD. Yet this very style of hers acted somewhat like a carrot drawing her forward toward the hope of winning her race to happiness by touching base with her ADD potential, a capacity she hasn't been able to utilize satisfactorily.

Ironically, the side of Nadine that needed the primary nurturing could not connect with the "Deep Thinker," who may have reflected an undeveloped, insufficiently educated, cognitive intelligence that added to her fragmentation. Almost as if validating this thought, she finished the discussion reflecting back on her interview for the elder-care job one-and-a-half years earlier, by saying, "They actually said in the [job] description that . . . the goal is to have their clients be happy and achieve their dreams!" Having said that, she gently exclaimed, "Oh my gosh, when one approaches life in the right way [for us with ADD], doors open."

Though she didn't get the job, she has held the remark within as a comfort for what might have been. And, if the medication for her bipolar disorder continues to help her remain balanced, perhaps she will have another chance.

YOUR TIME TO EMBRACE THE *TRUE YOU*

Nine Lives and a GPS Have Nothing on You

Regardless of how old you are, you always have time to find that wonderful, Waiting-in-the-Wings part of you called the *True You*. Cats have nothing on us. They only have nine lives. Each of us has as many lives as we are willing to work to create.

What's really good about this situation is that it puts the power in our hands to be how and what we want to be. Feel your Sense of Powerfulness and know that no one has a strategic plan on their drawing board that is right for you. Only *you* have the power and creativity to discover your own Inner Self that will manifest into the *True You* with the aid of your own personal nurturing. Thank goodness you've consistently been doing your growing and healing of woundedness throughout this book so that you can arrive at the end of this chapter with the cards stacked in your favor.

Now, mind you, finding the *True You* is not a totally static proposition. It is a process that never totally ends. But all the changes and variation along the way are moving toward the complete vision of the very best of what feels right for you.

You've been considering your timing, collecting experiences, following suggestions, and practicing basic skills. You've let yourself dream. You've used trial and error to discover what you were drawn toward energized by anticipation. And you've applied the brakes on further progress when you felt hesitation at proceeding further in the direction that you had been headed.

How cool to carry around your own personal GPS system within yourself that is activated by the wonderful ADD attribute of sensitivity. You've learned to be self-serving at no one else's expense—because anything else only drowns both the other person and yourself. With the *True You* intact, you both will survive.

Sure, you have to sacrifice along the way, but only your fears and doubts and wounded feelings. In their place, you'll pick up right timing to arrive at your destination at the perfect right time. Even hindrances and barricades, blocks and *shoulds* will only delay you for as long as is needed to make your true goals come out right in the end.

Mr. Critic has been put to rest and right paths have been chosen over wrong paths as you've come into the homestretch of the current leg of your life. Left behind are the "I wish I'd done its" coated in remorse. Instead, congratulate yourself and know that you will have achieved All the Things your *True You* of this Time in Your Life Wants Plus a Hundred Hundred More!

Now let us finish working together to protect what you've achieved so far by discovering the Accommodating You—the part of you that will protect what you've accomplished while further building and strengthening accommodations to the Analogue Attributes that make you what you are as you move into the world at large.

As you meet up with the Linear culture that surrounds all of us and as we team with our Linear colleagues and loved ones, we'll be clear about the value we bring to the table while honoring and appreciating what others bring from their Linear storehouse.

In the long run, we and they will be a mighty force to behold: one that brings the diversity of wholeness to bear for the good of all.

6

THE ACCOMMODATING YOU

The "Accommodating You" is the part of you that is critically important following the evolution, through hard work, of identifying your *True You*. Without it, your *True You* is vulnerable to being eroded and even lost or, at least, wounded when you put your work out into a culture that is not made for your natural brainstyle.

We all remain vulnerable to wounding that hasn't finished healing prior to the discovery and identity of our *True Self*. When this happens, aspects of new wounding may manifest, disrupting your ability to live fully and as wholly as is possible for your *True Self*, utilizing your skills, talents, and all that is special about yourself.

Fortunately, we can identify and teach another part of ourselves to protect and discover alternative ways to do what is needed without being further wounded as we take our *True Selves* out into the world. The name of the part is the Accommodating You.

I think of the Accommodating You as a rehab trainer that strengthens and protects the unwarped, unjudged, unwounded (or healed) natural you. Original innate skills, talents, attributes, and gifts with which you were born are available to you as you choose:

- To use them in order to accomplish any goal(s) you desire
- To reflect the way(s) in which your *True You* does business until wounding interferes
- To protect yourself by inventing alternative means to achieve a goal that is not a good *fit* for your ADD style of brain construction.

Unprotected and not properly prepared to mitigate problematic situations, you can again be led to becoming separated from using and enjoying the natural way in which you were made.

Without the protection of the Accommodating You, your vulnerability quotient rises. To the degree that you are doing something that doesn't *fit* or have been trying to achieve work in a non-ADD way, you will regress in your healing or incur new wounding. Such hurtful intrusion disregards your natural resources for learning and accomplishing things in your *True You* way. No wonder your progress is threatened. It may even take a nose dive underground, out of your conscious awareness.

But all is not lost when you understand the nature of Secondary Wounding that happens when ADD is not recognized for what it is: a natural style of brain construction that too often is misunderstood, leaving us in untenable situations that disempower and seriously wound us as a result.

WOUNDING AND SECONDARY WOUNDING CAN LEAD TO HEALING: ONE WOMAN'S ODYSSEY

Wounding and Secondary Wounding occur when you are under pressure to do something that isn't good for you and that isn't a natural *fit*. For example, after being identified with ADD, Mari (chapter 3) began to understand the wounding that she had suffered as a telephone customer service person. Conscientious, Mari stayed at that job for five years. In retrospect, she was able to describe how she felt during that time.

"I felt like a caged animal: sitting in that tiny cubicle, tethered to a telephone with no human contact, and providing the same 'scripted' answers day after day. I was utterly miserable."

The Secondary Wounding that she received as a result of the telemarketing job occurred because the lack of identification of her ADD brainstyle lowered her self-worth and created long-lasting depression. Required to do a job that didn't *fit* her led to Secondary Wounding that happens when she was put in an untenable situation because of her natural brainstyle.

Textbook in nature, here's the rest of Mari's story. "I suffered with clinical depression for years. Last year while I was on disability and in intense therapy, the doctors thought I might have bipolar disorder also. While in therapy, I did mention that a family physician said I was 'hyperactive' as a child. Also, a psychiatrist suspected the same thing years later when I had been in college. Since there was no course of treatment for ADD at the time, those doctors focused on the depression."

It was only last year that her current doctors evaluated her history more closely and decided that her depression was caused by traumatic events (probably what is being called Chronic Stress Disorder in this book). Armed with that information, she decided to make a closer study of how to cope with ADD. It was at that point that she found my book *ADD on the Job* and says it has also eased her depression.

"I realized I was working in an environment that was completely wrong for me, and that's why I was constantly stressed out and suicidal."

Awareness of wounding created her first major accommodation. Thus being misidentified with depression as the source of her problems created its own set of emotional problems that neither she nor professionals could remedy until the cause of the problem was properly identified. But when it was, oh my, how nice.

GOING BEYOND WOUNDING TO FORGIVENESS: A POWERFUL TOOL TO HEALING

To the degree to which you have gone through something like Mari, whose environment was totally toxic to her, you will have been wounded, too. If you haven't worked on the healing of this/ these experience(s), you must do it now to clear the path for the Accommodating You to function.

Hurt and frustrated, you may come to the conclusion that your *True You* dreams were nothing but fantasy. Grief may tear at you, accompanied by anger, depression, and even shame at seeming to have trusted in something, your dreams, that you innocently believed in to no avail.

But, stop right there! You're only experiencing a standard grief reaction. That's normal. Sure it hurts. However, it's not permanent nor does it mean that your bond to your dreams and your *True You* is severed. You have not lost everything. You have only gone astray through no fault of your own. So, let's get back on the path to ADD health.

This is where the enormous value of Accommodation comes into play both to encourage additional healing and also to learn to not be seduced into falling into a similar trap again, thus preserving and protecting your *True You* environment.

But before you move forward, there is one psychologically based move you need to take—the Act of Forgiveness. I'm not talking about a religious ritual. I'm speaking of a therapeutically powerful tool that can free you of the hurt and anger that you have carried.

When we are hurt or threatened in any way, we suffer a loss of safety. We grieve, which means we experience a grief reaction. We go into denial, get angry, feel guilty as we try to bargain our way out of the loss and become depressed. This series of emotional responses is trying to protect us from feeling our wounding.

Before we can finish the grief process of our dreams, so that we can accept whatever we think we've lost, we must forgive: mostly ourselves, but others, too, whom we think blocked us from reaching our goal, including our ADD, or Linear teachers, or parents.

It's time to FORGIVE YOURSELF and OTHERS knowing that you're already in the process of embracing your ADD and will learn how to find the environment that *fits* you.

Forgiveness Time is Now

Following forgiveness, there is a free path open for the Accommodating You to find the environment that is right for you and your wonderful ADD skills. One of the best ways to implement the forgiveness is to talk with another person who has an ADD brainstyle and has moved through the forgiveness phase of healing. You will see, in action, how to feel good about yourself.

You will come to understand that those who didn't know the truth about ADD had no way to know what to do to help you. It's almost like a miracle to find out that there isn't, and hasn't, been anything *wrong* with you all this time. It's more like a misunderstanding, like our ancestors thinking the world was flat or a particular race of people were subhuman.

When the insight strikes you, you will suddenly know the truth and can accept the congratulations you are due.

Please be aware that if you're unable to let go of your anger, depression, or hurt, it's because emotionally you still have some unfinished healing to do. A mental health counselor can be very helpful at this point, if you get stuck in the grief process. You deserve to get the help that will free you to be You. Then you can move on and embrace your *True You*.

THE ACCOMMODATING YOU GOES TO WORK

When you bring the Accommodating You to bear on your dreams, you may think of it as a tool that will connect you to success.

To accomplish your goal, you must be aware that:

- Other people's brainstyles affect everything they do—their ways of thinking, expressing, and acting—just as your brainstyle affects every part of you.
- The diversity of people's brainstyles also shapes the environments in which you will work, even if the people aren't there. You'll experience the effects, from the kinds of chairs to the very organization of the office in which you work. You will see a reflection of those who designed them.
- Products, instruments, and input that you absorb as you do your job will reflect various brainstyles, some of which will fit you and some that won't.
- The skills and education you need to learn for success—the required proposals and sales products that are required of you in order to even be heard, and the many, many ways in which doors open to us in our culture or remain closed—are all based on the match between your style of brain construction and that which you confront from outside of yourself.

I encourage you to simply be aware of your environment in relation to your brainstyle and trust your feelings to determine the accuracy of fit between your brainstyle and that associated with others you come in contact with and with the environment in which you will be functioning.

I discovered that I did better being self-employed because of my enormous sensitivity to *fit*. A couple of times, early in my career, I quit situations that made me feel depressed and rather crazy. I learned my lesson from these exchanges—as Mari did from her telephone customer service job. I simply could not, would not do anything for very long that I didn't agree was the right thing for me, as defined by how well it *fit* me.

Until you refine your accommodations to your ADD attributes, especially to your sensitivity to *fit*, you may find working with a mentor or counselor a valuable resource. You deserve to get the best education you can in reading what works for you and what to do about it.

ACCOMMODATION IN ACTION

Having prepared a way to improve the odds that you and your ADD style of brain construction can work to your advantage, let's look at specifics that you can draw upon to help you successfully accommodate the *True You*. Here are a few signs that you can carry in your billfold or hang on your wall:

There is nothing fundamentally wrong with me.
I deserve to succeed.

Watch Out!
For resistance you confront.
For discounts of you and your ways.
For what others think or say about you.

Words may lead you to feel inferior.
Labels wound as surely as fists.

Calmly speak up, letting others know
what you want and how to address you.

Build your emotional powerfulness.
Pull courage from within yourself.
Refuse to accept what you do not wish to receive.

Reach out to those of us who are not afraid
of brainstyle diversity.
Use us mentors as models as you strive to safeguard the *True You*,
while healing the Wounded You as you entice an imperfect world.

Skill-Building, Great and Small

There are as many "tips," "accommodations," and stories about how to improve your ADD-designed life as there are bits of sand on a beach. Both are ever-changing, adapting to the environment, and moving to and fro.

In this book, some will work for you, some will make you think of others, some of which will be of your own making, and some won't work for you. I trust your judgment about which ones to use and which to toss.

One Man's Pathway to Healing and Accommodation

You met Henry in chapter 2 of this book. First he told you about his background and what went wrong. Now he is ready to finish the rest of his story on a hopeful, calm journey to living out his *True Self*. You've already heard how he got into trouble. Now you'll hear what he's doing to get out of trouble so he can utilize the special skills of his ADD brainstyle.

After Henry lost the contract that fed his business, he was arrested. From there he ended up losing everything. At that point he turned a corner, becoming introspective.

In Henry's own words, he said, "I was propelled to take stock, which led me to finding a therapist who discovered my style of brain construction. I sought help to understand what happened, to change how I was, and to develop coping abilities."

Now he's on a great "be careful" track and starting to learn how to change. He's on his way to Self-Control. Here's the rest of Henry's story:

"First and foremost," Henry says, "I went into Recovery. With that mind-set and guidance directing me, I'm learning to accomplish a lot of things.

"I've learned to acknowledge my ADD attributes. Every day I learn something new about what it means to be Analogue and what I can do about it. And, I want to help others when I am ready. There's no rush, though, because I'm not rushing ever again. I need to reach stability in my life before I distract myself prematurely away from me and my kid. I remind myself that, I'm a work in progress and always will be."

There are choices of all sizes that he is making to stabilize himself: losing weight, becoming involved in acting and tennis, giving up drinking, refinding his faith, and—last but not least—learning about ADD.

Each of these steps is bringing a new perspective to Henry— honing a skill or reminding him of the need to balance his body, mind, spirit, and way of life. This takes time.

As Henry and I have been dialoguing over a period of nearly a year, he has continued to share insights, make growth steps, and definitely own his part in the use of poor judgment, often taking more responsibility for what he did or didn't do than he had the capability to manage at the time.

For example, the acting class has slowly brought him out from behind his psychological armor. Though making a slow start, he succeeded at becoming involved, thanks to the teacher's support and patience. Henry quickly noticed that about fifteen of the twenty people in the class were ADD. It helped him feel that he was with like-kind. It was hard, but then he said, "I just got up there and 'did it.' I knew that I would be accepted and understood and I felt safe for the first time in my life."

Finding my books on the Internet propelled him to write me an email. He had sufficient trust to do that. And better yet, he remained patient when I didn't respond right away, tardy as I was from recovering from a knee replacement. But when I got back to him, he was ready and open. More of his armor disintegrated. I've noticed that he is not in a rush, which affirms his perspective of his recovery.

Doing His Part

Using self-awareness and willingness to continue to consider outside guidance and help, Henry is attending to what are priorities in the cleanup of his past behavior: cleanup of ADD attributes gone wrong, cleanup of family aspects gone wrong (unintended as they were), cleanup for what might have helped him growing up but wouldn't get him where he wanted to go as an adult.

Of course he has to assume responsibility at the present—and that he is doing. But what he has to understand and correct is how and what went wrong in the first place. That child/teen/young adult will ultimately need to be forgiven by Henry for what he didn't know then.

What he desires, by letting me share his story, is that perhaps others can learn from what he now knows, before it is too late for them. His goal for himself is to find a path that will lead him in a healthy, fulfilling way to live with his *True Self*.

What Henry wants you to know about his discovery of his innate ADD brainstyle starts with the issue of his lack of ability to self-structure.

Henry says, "I overcompensated for my lack of structure with what I did well: sales. For a time, I didn't miss the lack of structure. I just made more sales to fill in the lack of structure.

"My talents as a sales person, negotiator, and leader led me to fast growth. I needed my talents supported, not disparaged. I needed to be told by the people with whom I worked that my wonderful talents and skills were doing the job. Thus, the protecting person would be giving me reasons to feel good about myself because of what I did well.

"Unfortunately, it was the things I didn't do well that would eventually sink my ship. And that is what my employees wanted to tell me about. But I didn't want to hear anything that I couldn't do because it made my feelings of inadequacy feel even worse."

This is a critical element in helping or trying to advise anyone with ADD. None of us can be "talked at" or criticized without experiencing brutal pain that shuts down our receptive systems. That's our sensitivity working overtime. And despite what is said by people who don't have the raw ADD sensitivity, it is simply not something that can be blown off. "Ignore it" and "Listen" said in a raised voice impairs the ADD person more. The result can be total shutdown—shutdown that is not planned, but happens with overwhelming feelings of helplessness that pull us down into a pit of blackness, or a total blind runaway, literally, from the situation.

Considering Henry's lack of innate structural skills, he's making headway thanks to input from the therapy and group help he is getting. Henry was able to say, "I built the business too quickly and so lost track of the proper planning steps—steps I'd never learned to put in place in my early life. Sure, my reading tutor came up with the 'tools' that I needed to move forward in elementary school, but the process of developing my own tools and steps from there on out didn't happen. I was bright enough to get by without learning how to work."

He avoided learning the Linear way of structuring his thinking in order to reach a goal and was not exposed to an Analogue way of structuring. His ability to interface with the world around him using structure that *fits* him will allow him to avoid additional wounding once he's developed Analogue structuring tools so he can protect his *True Self*. One of the best ways will be to work alongside someone who has the skills he needs to learn, so he can serve an unofficial apprenticeship. That way, he will learn.

He's learning that being himself is okay and that he doesn't have to be like anyone else—namely the model student in school or the "successful" adult male. Henry is beginning to feel his own "presence." When I asked him what this meant, he said, "I feel more real than ever before. Instead of playing a role, like in theater, I feel that I'm *me*. I'm not quite sure that I'm making sense—but yet, my feelings tell me I'm saying the right thing. I trust them.

"I've come to realize that because I could accomplish school work early on, yet couldn't do it in the 'right' way, I didn't connect with a solid sense of myself. Was I the 'one who got the answer?' Or was I 'the one who couldn't get the answer in the right way?'"

Considering that consistency is essential to stability (Core Components of Human Nature, chapter 2, p. 41), his social-emotional development languished. Because of his unidentified Analogue processing needs, he failed to develop a Sense of Trust that his needs would get met. His True childhood Identity, feelings of Competence, Powerfulness, and Self-Control were compromised. No wonder he bounced around needing to use a trial-and-error method of building a life.

Henry has shared an overview of who he was and is becoming. You will have your own story, as each of us does. And you and I and all of us are also "Works in Progress."

To achieve what we can on our journey into the world that surrounds us, we will need to be true to ourselves as we watch, listen, and learn who we are in the context of the dreams we hold in our hearts and the environments in which we move. We must protect against wounding, ever staying true to ourselves. In that way, we can contribute the best we have within us to our community at large. And, hopefully, those who are different from us will do the same. Together we will make up balanced teams of diversity where we are all valued for how we are.

To the end of strengthening the identification and use of our ADD attributes, the rest of this chapter will reflect some of the myriad Analogue contributions that we can honor within ourselves and share with the world in which we live.

FINDING AND PROTECTING THE BRAINSTYLE THAT WORKS FOR YOU

In business, perhaps you work for a company that tracks sales income and expenditures monthly. Every month leaves you in the worst possible muddle. You have no way of recalling where you put all the notes and slips of paper you made every day of the month. Mileage? The extra sale to a customer in a nearby town eludes you. The business lunch you paid cash for, where is the receipt?

It usually takes you a whole weekend of stress and pain to fill in the required forms and the job you do is usually not very accurate. Being honest by nature, you usually shortchange yourself.

Your company is not run by "bad guys." The board of directors has spent money on respected notebook guides in which you can track your financial dealings on a daily basis and then transfer the figure to a sheet that is sort of like using the back of a bank statement. There are even directions to guide you through the process of figuring out your sums.

But the problem is that you have to fill in the forms. In the throes of work, immersed in your job, talking to people, opening new contacts, and making sales and courtesy calls to customers of long standing, you forget to record the data into your financial guide. Or you're doing a favor for a customer or following up on something that a colleague needs. Or you write down the wrong number even when you try really hard to be accurate. You never know how you get distracted. You are so much more people oriented than paper oriented that the paper work simply doesn't get done. You mean to do it. You try. You make New Year's resolutions. You promise your boss you'll get it done. But, woe is you.

No wonder your bookkeeping is a muddle at the end of the month. Your spouse is fed up with having to listen to you complaining one weekend a month while you're holed up in the den so the kids have to rely on only one parent for everything. She tries to help you, but without the daily numbers, there's no hope. And besides, you always end up fighting about your not having done it.

You got an iPhone, to remind you daily, but that didn't work. You just turned the reminder alarm way down so that it wouldn't interrupt you when you were with a client. Your spouse even reminds you in the morning, but as soon as you're on the road, you forget whatever she was reminding you of.

Why does all of this happen?

It happens because your wonderful ADD style of brain construction doesn't track things in the way that non-ADD, Linear brains do. Both have systems that work. But the natural systems are totally different from one another. And because our culture tends to use a Linear system for tracking and organizing most things, we're taught in a Linear mode starting as a young child—all the time having an alternative way of structuring and organizing that would work better if that is how we are constructed. The end result is that we never develop our natural style for doing things and the result is the massive muddle you just read about.

We've already discussed our positive natural Analogue attributes. Now we are going to retrieve that list, practice it, and learn to feel good about the way in which we are constructed. Let's build your repertoire of skills:

Big Picture Viewing
How Things Function
Patterns and Relationships
High Levels of Activity
Kinesthetic Learning
Inner Locus of Control
High Sensitivity
Strong Sensing Capability
Organic/Rhythmic Movement

ACCOMMODATION TOOLS WE HAVE
TO WORK WITH

Each of these attributes may be applied to help us to structure projects in which we take part. Let's begin applying them to a difficulty faced by a lot of ADD/ADHD people who experience trouble structuring work, life, time, and most anything.

Big Picture Structuring and Organizing

I'm as outspoken as I am because I've gone through anger at being denied respect to a place of focusing on what is good about ADD attributes so we can use them to advantage. Watching the incredible transition that has occurred when we join forces with our natural attributes brings peace to my heart and a smile to my face.

So, with these warm thoughts, we will focus on accommodating the discrepancies between our Analogue brainstyle and the Linear culture in which we find ourselves so we can work in the best interest of our *True Selves*. Let's start by considering how we can structure a project, goal, or assignment using our Analogue processing brains.

A key ADD attribute that works well for us is the way in which we first see the Big Picture of the end goal. This happens before we can make plans or understand how to create or implement the goal or project.

Usually creative by nature, Big Picture people often see a complete vision of what we want to achieve before we start moving toward any goals. In fact, we don't travel well to any goal unless we *are* provided with the Big Picture to begin with.

Choose a project that you want to structure. It can be anything in the world that you'd like to work with—from a relationship to a new business, such as Henry did in chapter 2, p. 71. Perhaps it's a book you want to write or a child's birthday party you want to give. You may wish to start the business you've always dreamed of owning or create the dream you always wanted to manifest.

Begin by journaling or dialoguing about your thoughts and ideas—thoughts and ideas that have refused to go away no matter what you did. Keep your responses simple to begin with. Feel free to dream liberally. Jot down all the bits and pieces of ideas that come to mind. I don't expect you to do the whole job in one sitting. I just want you to begin a process that captures the elements that make up your dream.

Now commit to putting in writing, what you'd like to start producing.

I'd like to work on <u>(insert a project you'd like to do)</u>

Here are some thoughts to consider in order to begin the creation of your project: As an ADD person, you are likely to see the finished product instantly. This is your Big Picture attribute that has to be considered before you can effectively create your dream or manifest your idea. Basically, you'll have a lot of thoughts and feelings that are fragmented at first.

As long as three decades ago, I realized that I would see in my mind's eye a jumble of visual fragments, thoughts, feelings, and incomplete bits and pieces of information on the left side of my mind, and the Big Picture on the far right side of my mind. I wondered how to get from the left to the right. You see, there was nothing but blackness in between the two sides.

It didn't take me long to realize that was why I always had such a hard time implementing a goal—because I couldn't figure out what the steps were to get from the *idea* to the *formation* of the project. I'd been endlessly taught to make Linear steps in order to outline how to proceed, but to no avail. That just didn't work for me. I would always end up messing around until I finally achieved a suitable outcome. The outcomes were usually acceptable and adequate or better. But I felt guilty because I didn't achieve them in "the right way."

I knew there were steps. But for me, I simply couldn't figure out what to do to get from one place to another—not until I realized that I needed to start with the Goal Picture and bring forth the *function* of the goal before I could have any hope to build the end product. The going was, and still is, slow. It takes me several or many trials, experimenting with different combinations, before I find the one that begins to sing to me.

But I've discovered that the more I immerse myself in the function the product will serve, and give myself permission to shuffle pieces in and out of line, the sooner pieces will begin to fit together. I must experiment hands on. This may mean talking out loud about what I'm doing or using trial and error to achieve a step. Suddenly I begin to see parts of the building pattern. It does me no good to read about it.

Instead, the individual details tend to have a life of their own as if they are heat-seeking missiles that target where to go in order to achieve the outcome demanded by the function. I learned to trust to let this happen in order to form a pattern that would produce the product that would serve me and those who would be interested in the outcome.

You will see your potential model that is your dream, and that you can keep in mind to see whether you're going in the direction that you want if, in fact, you decide your next step *only* after you finish the previous step.

If you are primarily an Analogue processor, trying to use a Linear approach may start making you feel "crazy," stressed, and/or muddled. For this book, I trusted my Nonlinear approach. I didn't proceed to the writing of the *True You* chapter until I'd written about the prison-work insight that ADD symptoms were really symptoms of *fit* rather than symptoms of a brainstyle. That was the key—and after that, the rest of the book fell in place.

I doubt that I am the only one who has ever had this experience. You and I probably have tended to add to our poor feelings about ourselves, collecting experiences to inflate our Chronic Stress Response (CSR). So many of us quit at this time, giving up not just the ability to improve our writing through help from others, but giving up expression of our dreams, hopes, and passions. The trick is to find someone who will help you use the style of brain construction that naturally fits you.

Has this happened to you? Do you think and fear you are not talented or smart enough to accomplish the task? For what it's worth, you need to rethink your observation of yourself, because what happened to you had nothing to do with your talent, IQ, or capability. It had to do with an incorrect belief that all people learn and work in the same way.

Stake out your territory and follow your own way to use your talents and gifts—ways that *fit* you.

You are likely to have a very creative idea—one that is truly original or quite wonderful, one that is a very good idea. You may find that organizing in Big Picture ways works for you. It also means that you will have to find small pieces of the Big Picture that are alike and differentiate them from the whole. Pairing up with like-kind, finding someone whose brainstyle is similar to yours is likely to give you the road map for early steps to take, followed by later steps and, finally, finishing steps. What you will have accomplished is an apprenticeship— the teacher/learning model that works best for you.

In addition, do not hesitate to pair up with a counterpart who is a Bridge person who can help you connect with your goals. My editor on this project has been that sort of person. In my earlier professional life, I attribute a lot of my success to having had an office manager and secretary who used their skills to help me reach the career goals that I could not access alone.

Caution: Where the Big Picture Can Cause You Trouble

You may take on more than you can hope to chew over time. You may build a structure, like Henry, that doesn't have infrastructure to hold all the aspects of the project together in a way that is necessary for success.

It's not that Henry used a Big Picture approach that caused him trouble. It's that he left pieces out that needed to be there, and couldn't listen to input from people who knew what was needed.

It's also that your emotional engine may get revved too high. Too excited, you need balancing along the way.

The Gifts That You Offer Your Project

The gifts that you offer to the project may be your expansive thinking and perception, your creativity, and your ability to contribute these and other aspects of yourself so that eventually you and your gifts fulfill some specific role or goal with purpose that means success will be the outcome.

Let's say that you have a special talent that your project depends upon. For example it may be your athletic prowess, artistic talent, scientific inquiry skills, memory, salesmanship, leadership, money management, design capability, networking proficiency, or ability to read other people, etc. Write down what the special talents are that you bring to your project.

Let's investigate what you have to offer, and don't think that you aren't talented enough. Just put down what you love to do.

Special talents

_____

_____

What talents and skills do you especially wish to utilize:

_____

Next, I want you to list skills (not talents) that you know are needed in the business you're considering—such as financial planning, bookkeeping, logistics, human resources, and management skills—that you don't have:

_____

_____

If you don't have one of these skills do you know someone who
you trust who does? Also might the person be committed to you?
Might the person be available to join you in your undertaking?
Special trusted other(s):

_____

_____

How willing and able are you to seek help in arenas where you are
vulnerable, such as bookkeeping or marketing or . . . ? Be honest.
Will you give up control of parts of the project to someone else so
you can gain the input of a skill or talent you don't have? Do you
have money to pay someone to help you? Would you be willing to
give up part of the business in trade for a skill you don't have: How
willing are you to share your dream?

_____

_____

Whom do you think you might ask?

_____

_____

How might you find someone to help you if you don't know of
anyone?

_____

_____

I recommend that you play with these ideas, get together with
others who think the way you do and use the same language as
you do, but who have more experience than you do. You need a
mentor or mentors. Be aware of trying to use someone with Linear
thinking to mentor you. It usually doesn't work. Nor would it work
for you or any Analogue person to mentor them.

How Things Function

Another attribute of people with an ADD style of brain construction is to think in terms of how things function. If you are to know how to proceed toward a goal, you must know its purpose. How is this goal to be used? Rather than seeing the details that make up the task, you need to see the function the details play. Then you can know the steps to take to achieve the goal. Consider that details and steps are not synonymous for us.

Function is the player that we will talk about in relation to structuring and organizing what you want to do. The way you use it or the degree to which you utilize your strong ability to consider the function of things will depend on the type of project.

You ask, "How will I know how much attention I need or want to pay to my project, using my Function attribute?" That is not something you need to worry about. You will draw upon what you need whether you realize you do or not. If you want to be conscious of when you are thinking in terms of how something functions, all you have to do is ask yourself—and then, "don't try to think about it." Just observe and feel what you automatically think about and do.

Taking into account how something functions is a process. It's mobile. Looking at the Big Picture is more likely to yield a static picture initially, whereas a functional attribute has a sense of movement or motion embedded in it. So, to progress with Analogue structuring of anything, you will automatically mix the attribute of function into any idea or goal that comes to mind.

To do this, fill in the blanks below. Keep your responses simple. If you get enthusiastic about something you're thinking or seeing in your mind's eye, consider journaling about it separately from your project. That then becomes a purposeful "getting off track," which means you're still in control.

Considering how something that you're interested in may be influenced by its function can be heady stuff. So get ready to have some fun. Let's say you are thinking of how to invent a new approach to using something that you know a lot about. It could be a program, a service, an economic relationship, a chemical process with a new outcome that would benefit a lot of people, a new set of laws that would rule a sporting event, how illnesses can develop as a function of stress, and on and on

My interest is: _____

_____

A function implies there will be a definite end to the application of that function, or a particular kind of way of achieving the process involved. The outgrowth may imply a whole new relationship. So see what pops up in your mind. Do you see particular people coming to mind: colleagues, work buddies, volunteer friends, parents with children the same age as yours?

What are you feeling as you consider something in your life that you are doing and want to change, or something that really irritates you the way it is structured or organized, so much so that you'd like to create a different way for it to function?

One of my friends is drawn to working in the arena of disaster management. As she edges toward following her *True Self*, she can spend time dreaming, journaling, and talking about ideas that will serve the function of working with behavior management. Next, she can develop relationships, discover information, and make plans for what she's thinking about doing and will begin to have an idea of a place to start. After that, she'll be better able to see whether she still likes the idea of work in the disaster field.

Your job now is to consider further whether you have something you'd like to improve. It could be something you'd like see improved because you don't like the way it is run. You might want to help improve a service or organization so that it could be more functional. Describe a situation that comes to mind, including your ideas for improvement. (If you feel stuck, start by recalling the last few complaints that you voiced):

_____

_____

_____

Use additional paper if needed.

As an Analogue thinking person, you may find yourself tracking down a number of blind alleys. Or maybe you have a plate of
spaghetti-ideas that are getting tangled up in your mind. Could be
that you have so many ideas that you are becoming confused and
ready to give up because you see no way to make a sensible decision.

Wisdoms

Important "wisdoms" that you can follow will guide you to
make decisions along the way.

- You don't need to follow up on every idea that comes to you.
- Set a limited time to let your mind drift, and then get up
  and mingle with people—be active, go grocery shopping, or
  do some other everyday aspect of life. This will help you get
  grounded again.
- Make a few notes, not in-depth at this early point, but to
  keep the topic on your list—oh yes, you're going to make a
  list of things that you are thinking about.
- Give yourself a week or two during which you update your
  notes, not by writing reams of notes but short notes.
- At the end of this time, review your notes and see how many
  times you have listed the same item on different days. Sometimes an idea will hound you. It just keeps coming back time
  after time after time. (Sometimes this will go on for months
  or years if you don't act on it.)
- Talk to a confidant or several people about your top five
  ideas. As you do, focus on how you feel about each idea.
  Spoken out loud, the idea may not sound as great as it did

in your head. Or it may sound even better than when you first came up with it. Never choose a skeptic to talk with. That will drag you down emotionally and is not good for your creativity.

- When you feel the pressure of being ready to act, say "I want to do something special." Then become alert to bodily sensations that reverberate throughout your mind and body, when you are in relationship to one of your ideas. This will lead you to commit to one idea, goal, or process.

- Most important: "IT DOESN'T MAKE ANY DIFFER-ENCE WHICH IDEA YOU CHOOSE OF YOUR TOP CANDIDATES AWAITING YOUR CHOICE." You must recognize this and honor it. Why?

- Because no matter which project you choose, you will be the one conceiving it and the one responsible for playing it out. Any idea will have your stamp on it, so any idea will turn out okay. You will cast your choice in your own mold and it will show your strengths and your weaknesses.

- If you have chosen one and feel okay about the one you've chosen, set the others aside. In the future, one or more of them may have endured and you can return later to give that idea its turn. If not, it wasn't meant to be, and you will have given your best shot to having given one of your ideas the benefit of your interest and attributes.

Caution: Where the Functional Approach Can Cause You Trouble

The biggest issue that can go wrong when you're using the functional approach is to fail to believe in yourself. If you try to dream, make choices, and activate a choice that you think you *should* do, you will have set yourself up for heartache and you won't be following your own inner truth.

Proceeding to a goal, we must know our purpose. If the purpose is only self-serving or is used to garner approval from someone else, again, you are danger of not having the full support of your heart and emotional system. Too often, our conscious mind makes decisions based on *wrong* reasons for what the *True You* wants.

Let's say a parent believes that success depends on achieving professional status in the culture. You might be able to achieve the role, but what if you really wanted to be an artist?

One woman I knew earned a PhD in microbiology at a top school at the urging of her parents. She wanted, in fact, to be an artist, and she had an artist's talents and a creative ADD brainstyle, but did not have the emotional powerfulness as a young adult to go against her parent's wishes to pursue her own goals.

As a result, she suffered from depression and ill health for years until she finally discovered the reason. She really wanted to make beautiful things that in her thinking would make the world a better place. She felt her life was filled with worthless drudgery and her heart was breaking as she failed to fulfill her creative desires. Finally, the function of her life's path was realized fulfilling her core being. She quit her laboratory job and became self-employed as an artist. And she became a happy, healthy middle-aged woman.

Structuring By Virtue of Patterns and Relationships

One of the biggest tools we have to work with as Analogue processors is our ability to pay attention to the patterns and relationships within the Big Picture. One of the historic diagnostic criteria for Attention Deficit Disorder is a lack of attention. The problem with using that as a "symptom " of ADD is that it doesn't define what is to be attended to. In reality we have incredible attention when it comes to seeing the Big Picture, the patterns and relationships between people and things, how things function, and when we are working kinesthetically.

Were your parents told that you didn't pay attention in class? Were you accused of daydreaming as you gazed out the window?

It was true that you had an Analogue brainstyle. But you certainly didn't have a problem with attention to patterns and relationships. Faced with even a small opportunity to learn in a kinesthetic way, you were an eager, attentive student. But faced with desk work, you shifted your attention to the Big Picture of the outside world and to the dreams that were in your head. You might even have been attending to ways in which you might use the lesson that you were being taught. It's possible that you understood the lesson and immediately went on to apply that lesson in your life. On that mental journey, you would likely find lots of interesting material to learn from, to pay attention to, and to create from.

Let us go back to the Big Picture with the many details scattered throughout the original picture. Do you recall some of the parts of the program? Rather than being seen as individually ordered items that fall in a straight line, they may have been seen by you and me as pairs and triads and groups that have a relationship to one another and that serve a function in the big scheme of things, the Big Picture. As the function of the groupings begins to be expressed, then the whole plan for the organization of the project also begins to fall in place.

With our focus of attention on the relationships between details rather than on the details themselves, we tend to glean more in-depth understanding of what's going on and of what can occur. Before long, if the project had to do with laying out a book, the designing of an airport, the running of an optometrist's office, or the planting of acres of farm land, the writer or architect, optometrist or farmer would have seen and organized the design plan having quickly seen the patterns and relationships from different aspects needed to reach a successful goal.

This would include overall design for flow of materials, services, personnel, and traffic—whether it be of words for the writer's book; runways at the airport; patient movement through the various screenings, prescription assessments, and treatment rooms for the optometrist and staff; placement of the barns and farm equipment in relation to the fields that needed to be plowed or left fallow so as not to exhaust the earth, or roadways for the harvesting of produce so it can efficiently be loaded for travel to its destinations.

Now to you . . . Is there an organizational problem that comes to your mind immediately to which you would like to apply a detailed analysis of patterning and relationships? It could be relative to people and their movement, between individuals or groups, or a pattern between objects or processes or beliefs, or . . . What do you come up with that has been a part of your life that you now understand the importance of recognizing the pattern(s) involved?

_____

_____

Of profound importance to me has been the emergence of the relationship that evolved between Attention Deficit Disorder and the concept of diversity. It wasn't until I began to see (in my mind) and feel that the history of African American culture in this country was very similar to the way people labeled with ADD had been identified and treated as having something *wrong* with them that the concept of diversity flew into my mind. Both were originally considered to be deficient, less than, or disordered. Oh, my goodness. Once that pattern emerged for me, there was no going back. I saw the pattern. I felt the pattern. I knew the pattern. What was I to do about what I saw? I needed to plan.

What about you? Think of relationships of situations or groups of people that you suddenly saw in a whole new light.

_____

_____

_____

Caution: Where Pattern and Relationship Focus Can Cause You Trouble

The biggest problem results from overlooking details that are essential to a Linear structure that is present as a backdrop. With a worker's attention so focused, even absorbed by the style of the creation, filing papers, crossing "t"s and dotting "i"s may be overlooked. Tempers may even rise when the love and attention to the patterning and relationships seems more important than some little bit of minutia.

Obviously both large and small, fluid and static, pattern and detail must be a part of the Big Picture. They are needed to accomplish the best of results. Up rears the head of teamwork, yet another time.

The Gift That You Offer Your Project

The really good news is that by being aware of the relationships and patterns in our projects, we often can work more quickly and efficiently than if we stayed on a detailed base level. Many times, there seems to be a personal touch that can be felt by those who become involved with the project of an Analogue worker/creator. It's sort of like being able to sink into the patterns, becoming a part of the process, having a relationship with the process.

High Levels of Activity Get a Lot of Everything Done, Physically, Mentally, Emotionally, and Verbally While Rhythm Greases the Wheels

Superficially, a high activity level seems to be so familiar to the ADD world that it may seem to have little bearing on serious, adult projects. When you're considering the effects activity may have on the organization and structuring of a project, you must consider the four activity arenas in which ADD attributes show up: physical, mental, emotional, and verbal.

Choose any project that you've already thought through and add High Activity Level to its making. You may, of course, choose a new project. Let's see how this affects what and how you tackle your project. What extra assets do you bring to the project, especially if you are ADHD?

The project I choose: _____

Now here are some questions to explore.

In the early phase of your project's creation, are you aware of the rapid processing of information mentally, the visions, or stage plays of your mind including the dialogue that you may hear? Do you remember the first stage of viewing the Big Picture of your project? As you scanned this early vision from the past in retrospect, did you tend to view much larger amounts of potential material than you later discovered you could, or needed to, include for a successful outcome? Or do you notice that you tended to visualize a minimalistic overview that you later expanded with more dimensions as you worked on developing the project?

In the beginning I viewed larger amounts of creative elements than I could use later on. _____ yes _____ no

In the beginning I started with a limited overview (somewhat bare bones) that I later filled in as I progressed. _____ yes _____ no

Either way is fine, but they are different. It behooves you to know how you work so that you keep tabs on a potential timetable that usually needs to be associated with the project.

We all have a natural sense of timing and rhythm that needs to be honored. (I tend to view a much bigger and jam-packed Big Picture than I may have time or money to create.) We may be in danger of setting ourselves up for "burnout" as we get tired of the project we chose as we attempted to finish it, because it grew beyond our bounds. We simply couldn't stay with it.

Time management is acutely associated with our activity level and the ups and downs of our energy to move forward consistently to an end. We are likely to swing from overwork to insufficient work time spent to complete the job. We must beware of boredom which creates mind-boggling depression material for many of us ADD folks and exhaustion that may lead us to the ER.

When you consider a new project, you may have noticed that your motivation is high. To be sure, you may have been accused of having "Newness Addiction," that is, seriously rushing to obtain or do something new, only to quickly lose interest once you've mastered the activity or learned all you can learn from the project. Repetition is not a friend of most people with an ADD brainstyle.

The good side of this tendency is that it "gets things started." The bad side might seem to be a tendency to drop the ball after a short time. Being kinesthetic learners, however, we tend to feel the project as we pursue it. Add to that our intense initial interaction with the project and the odds go up that we will know fairly quickly whether the project is going to hold our attention or not.

Had we worked more slowly on the initial entry into the project, it might have taken a good deal more time to figure out that the project wasn't that interesting for us. One more add-on is the fact that because we have intense and deep emotions, we may quickly get deeper into the meaning and understanding of the personality of the project and, again, learn more quickly that we are not as interested as we initially thought we would be. Well, that way we lose less of our lifetime on things that don't work out in the long run! (This could be a joke, but it also could be a very wise statement.)

The Popcorn Popping Model

Speaking of humor, a variation on starting and stopping behavior as you begin a project is what I've labeled the Popcorn Popping Method of Settling into a Day of Focused Work.

Here's what happens. I get up and move to my desk to begin to work for the day. I sit down, open my computer, and reach for my papers. Next thing I know, I get back up and go to the kitchen. Hmm, coffee or orange juice first? While I am deciding, I notice that the trash needs emptying, and so swoop down to do that, start the coffee, and pull a couple of things out of the refrigerator that

I might use to pack my lunch when I go the library to change my scenery later in the day. While I'm waiting for the coffee to drip, I sit back down at my desk and pull out several folders. Then I pop up again because the coffee is done and I need to foam some goat milk to put on top. Oh, I see I didn't finish washing all my dishes last night, so I do that and then sprinkle cinnamon on top of the coffee foam and go back to work.

Sitting down, I remember that I need to make a phone call. So I pop back up to get my appointment book out of my purse in the other room to confirm an appointment. Back at the desk, I make my call, get up to return my appointment book to my purse—everything has a place, a home where it lives so I know where to find what I need when I need it. I have enough trouble setting car keys and cell phone down on shelves such that I can't find them, so I'm very, very careful where I put things.

Back at the computer, I notice some new emails that have come through, so I glance at them, trash a couple, and make a note to follow up on a couple. Then I realize I'm getting cool, so I decide to get dressed to go out in a few hours. It's on my way to the bedroom that I see straight pins on the floor from last night's sewing. Better pick them up and put them down the hall in my sewing basket where they belong so no one steps on them! That reminds me that I'd planned to transfer my sewing to a new basket tonight or tomorrow. So while I'm in the closet, I pull the new basket down and put it next to the old one. Dressed, on my way back to start working at my desk, I discover I let my coffee set too long. I really, really dislike lukewarm coffee, so I grab the cup, set it in the microwave for a minute, decide to forgo more goat-milk foaming, and fold kitchen towels while waiting the interminable time a minute takes to pass while the coffee is warming. I prepare a glass of ice water to take back with me for after I finish drinking my hot coffee.

Nicely heated coffee, I turn to walk back to my desk when suddenly, I'm ready to work.

The light bulb goes off in my mind. I know where to start, I know what my whole day is going to look like, and I'm eager to write and make progress. My day's Big Picture has popped out of the Popcorn Processor and off I go.

Not only do I know what I'm going to write, I know that I'll stay seated now for an appreciable length of time.

I've noticed that if I force myself to stay seated with my initial confusion bumping around, whatever I write, I end up throwing out later in the day or the next day. I know that I won't be able to keep my mind on the content of my work while I'm drawn off to the need to warm my coffee and then have a glass of water with ice to drink as I want it. Perhaps it's like I got my physical exercise so I become ready to be still for an appreciable time.

Obviously, there is a connection between physical movement, in this case popping up and down, and the clarity of functioning of mind and the focusing of my attention. Once I'm "popped out," I wouldn't think of moving until I finished a segment that I was working on. Sometimes I have been on such a roll that I even work too long in the sense that I get overtired. I try not to do that. But it is a glorious feeling to finish a unit—a unit that has come together with great clarity of mind.

Self-Gratitude for My Way of Managing Me

My way of managing my activity level, organizational skills, and creativity *fits* me. The result is that I am able to do what I do as I want to do it, both in the way of process and in the content the work contains. And I promise, I've taught myself not to fight it.

Regardless of how your activity level marks the initial stage of work for organizational purposes, it is important to know how you are made and then plan for it. There is no reason to judge this behavior. That is a useless response.

Do you function at a Highly Activity level at the beginning of projects, activities, and new situations? _____ yes _____ no

If you answered "yes," let's think about the value of High Activity to your project organization and introduce Self-Control so you use the High Activity to advantage. You do not need to change, nor are you addictive. You simply are the way you are, so learn to use it constructively.

Time and Timing Skills

Think of yourself as the lead runner on a relay team. Become aware of how long you are likely to stay actively involved. Base your estimate on past experience and how you are feeling at the moment. Remember, no judgments. That may lead to a tendency to not quite be truthful with yourself.

Then figure out how long this project may interest you or how quickly you'd like to have it finished. Remember you're in control. You may wish to begin this analysis by considering the first stage in the project—try calling it "Startup" or "Exploration." Personally, I wouldn't try to analyze the whole project, but would tackle one or a few beginning stages. But that's me. If that feels "right" to you, try it the same way. If a different breaking point feels better to you, try your way. But be sure not to bite off too much to chew since it's important to have some success early on because you finished what you started—thus, small bits yield better results.

Although I love the ideas and concepts in this book and embrace the opportunity to communicate, I really don't like to write anything this long. I prefer to write short stories that may be done in one setting or an hour or two. With the latter, the project comes out all in one fell swoop. It's a whole unit from the beginning, even if I didn't realize it would be when I started. Out it comes in its entirety. Whereas a book like this actually has many books in it. The whole book ultimately needs to hang together, but I also will think of it as having "sections," spaces that can be created in shorter order.

The introductory stage of interviewing and writing people's stories helps motivate me because it tweaks my interest for three reasons. I like talking with people and I like writing stories. It's also an easy thing for me to do as it doesn't take any organizing. And, finally, I feel responsible to share the person's story with others, for both to gain from.

My job is to know how to maximize my time over the long haul. Actually, I'm pretty good with time and timing. It feels natural to me. But my ADD contributes to a need to move around frequently, so I honor that first because I can count on myself to be time aware and timely.

Henry, on the other hand, was different from me when it came to spending time on his work. His job in building his sales business was to realize that he was good for long periods of time during the initial startup phase of development when he was doing the kind of work that *fit* his style of brain construction. But he had little patience to spend time with something that *didn't fit* him.

Now as he heals the mess he made and factors in components other than sales and marketing—such as dealing with finances, logistics, personnel, and operations—he will be able to consider the amount of time involvement that he needs to put in doing what he does well. At that point, he must commit to a time plan that will see him to success, and that means turning the other aspects of the job over to other people with skills he does not have. He doesn't have to do everything. He only has to see that everything gets done in a timely manner.

Managing Your Energy

When you consider your ADD activity level and your ability to organize your time effectively, you have the resources you need to get your work done and take care of yourself. Physically, everyone has physical ups and downs throughout the day that remain relatively consistent over time. In order to maximize your time, you need to know what time of day you work best. There are morning people, and evening people, and dark-of-night people.

What time of day maximizes your energy?

_____

_____

I am a _____ -time person. Describe your daily cycle of energy by the hours when you are most alert and most dull or tired. Then do the best you can to factor that into your daily plan of action. Here's a schedule that I think would work for me:

_____

_____

I'm assuming that you're using common sense with your health so that you're not partying every night or drinking or taking drugs to manage your emotions or energy. You don't have to be a saint. Of course an occasional cutting loose (within sensible limits) is fine when you don't have work to do within hours of your playtime.

One trick that works really well for some people is a Power Nap. Again, some people can shut their eyes for a minute or two while others, if they nap in the daytime, upon awakening, are not able to function the rest of the day. You know who you are. Take advantage of your natural tendency without trying to be who you are not. Do what works for you. Take that responsibility.

Rhythm is important and a natural attribute that will help you manage your high activity level, be it mental or physical. Use it to relax, to move from one kind of work or activity to another, to calm down, to lie down to drift and dream to music or mental visions.

One great example is in housecleaning. Instead of pushing yourself to do a marathon pre-company cleaning that you at-tempt to do in a methodical way, consider choreographing a cleaning dance that moves back and forth between rooms. Sure you may use more time to pick something up in the kitchen and carry it to the bedroom, then get something from the bedroom that needs to go into the bathroom where you find the scouring powder, which reminds you that the kitchen sink needs cleaning, too. But if you move as a flowing dancer, you will end up not tired. And you'll have had good, relaxing exercise that will actually energize you—and you'll have your house cleaned.

Just remember to live organically, which means to me that you are in synch with nature and embrace the rhythms of yourself and your environment as well as the activities that you introduce into your life.

Emotional Activity

Emotional activity tends also to be variable. Our big, broad, expressive emotions both energize us and give us charisma that draws helpers and clients and customers to us. You must be sure that, when you are networking or communicating with others, your emotions are in good shape because they will speak louder than words. If you have emotional work to heal—such as anger, a temper, feelings of low self-esteem, and/or depression—you need to work with a counselor to help you get beyond the emotions. Otherwise, they will communicate loud and clear. Your charisma will turn into repellent. You deserve better than that.

If you were the victim of wounding because of your ADD sensitivity, work with that also. It may take counseling or, at least, mentorship with another ADD person who has "been there," and cleared a lot of the hurt. Until you do, you will be setting yourself up for disappointment. But you deserve to feel good, so do your emotional healing work and then get on to embrace the success your *True Self* desires and deserves.

Now consider a project or situation you want/need to organize and write the ways that you can use your high Activity Level to advantage.

_____

_____

_____

_____

_____

Use additional paper as needed.

Verbal Activity

Lastly, let us consider Verbal Activity. Talking through what you're thinking may be one of the greatest gifts you have. And, like the other forms of activity with which we are blessed, too much talking or talking over someone else or using talking to win power are not constructive.

You've heard the quip, "He (the salesman) could sell refrigerators to Eskimos." The problem is that when the person you've caught in your verbal net becomes aware that she or he doesn't need what you're selling, you've lost not just the next sale, but also a contact, thus weakening or destroying your network of potential contacts, as well as clients and referrals, too. Be sure to consider others even though you're eager to succeed at your sales job. This takes Self-Control, but you can do it.

Many of us have words, words, and more words. I tend to apologize a lot for adding "Color Commentary" into my conversations. Ask me a simple question and you're likely to get a story or a history lesson. It's entertaining, but sometimes the pained look on the face of my listener tells me to "zip it up." So I do. I may even apologize, a bit shame-faced. Being thoughtful goes a long way to preserving relationships even when we're chatterboxes.

The good news is that spontaneous improv is a "no brainer." Ask a question and you'll get an entertaining or empathetic response. Somewhat related, about thirty-five years ago, I realized that I got instantly smart as soon as I was asked a question: not a question that had only one right answer like in school, but a plain old question. And it's remained true ever since. I'd love to know the neuroscientific reason for this, but I suspect it just means that the smart part of my brain is where my wisdom and intelligence lies—not in my frontal lobes that are in charge of memorized learning, organization, and planning—but elsewhere.

Another irony that I've noticed has to do with learning from conversations. I've learned that if I simply talk about a subject, sooner or later I will speak a lot of ideas, concepts and even new perspectives that I never consciously was aware I knew.

I'll never forget the day in the 1970s when I was a presenter at a child care provider workshop for caregivers of three- to five-year olds. I'd been talking about the first four stages of the Core Components of Human Behavior (chapter 2). I didn't know what the fifth stage was, though I sensed that there was one and sensed it would be the final one.

As the last words about developing a Sense of Powerfulness left my mouth that day, the first words about Self-Control tumbled out. The words proclaimed the name of the stage followed by a complete description of the concept that completed the Core Components of Human Behavior theory of sociocultural development in preschool children. Subsequently, I've never found a reason to change what I spoke of that day. For several weeks, I had been trying to think what that final stage would look like. I recall walking up and down the hallway at another conference to no avail. The insight didn't come . . . until it came the day that it did come to me—like birthing a child in its own time.

Where did this come from, this learning material I didn't know that I knew? What a gift. It has continued to happen from time to time, usually less dramatically, but nonetheless equally valid and useful. I've learned to trust what I say and respect the teacher part of me that I can count on as I organize, structure, and create programs and solutions, in order to reach goals based on the gift of speaking I have been given.

Caution: Where Your High Activity Level Can Cause You Trouble

Consider physical, mental, emotional, and verbal activity levels. Despite all the assets brought by high activity levels, the biggest downside is that there is little room for poor mental health or poor impulse control. When high-speed driving gets out of control, it can endanger your well-being and even your life or the life and safety of others. Other high-risk physical activities include downhill skiing, race-car driving, off-road biking, horseback riding, etc. requiring skills beyond what you may have developed. Please remember that even driving too fast in a busy city or on a residential street can have dangerous outcomes. A car, after all, is a deadly weapon.

Overly high mental activity can unground you from everyday life, making you unbalanced so much so that you lose your common sense—usually a strong gift of many people with an ADD brainstyle. Don't forget to breathe . . . and I don't mean pant.

As Henry's mind raced and his behavior kept trying to fix things by running faster and faster while doing the same things that hadn't worked the day before, he more and more lost touch with the reality of his everyday loss, not seeing what was happening around him until his whole business imploded.

Emotional hyperactivity, uncontrolled, can turn into manic behavior in response to attempts to cover inner pain and fear. Without a level head and clear mind that is able to be turned off so you can relax, hyper behavior is a liability. However, despite some popular misconceptions, these symptoms per se are not attributes of ADD.

Kinesthetic Learning, Hands-On Activity at Its Best

When we have a lot of ADD attributes, we most surely will tend to be kinesthetic learners, which means we learn through the process of doing something rather than reading or listening about whatever we want to learn.

On a practical level, those of us with ADD attributes need to be taught through using our strong kinesthetic learning skills from which the apprenticeship method of education evolved. Since we can use our Analogue attributes to more easily learn most of what we need to learn, there is no reason to struggle through trying to learn in a way that doesn't fit us. It would be equally improper to expect students with Linear attributes to learn in a primarily Analogue system.

Of course there is some use to learning some of the skills that are not primary to us. But it makes no sense to walk uphill on our hands when we have perfectly good feet to do the job. Prior to standardized one-size-fits-all education, there were many people who made enormous contributions to our society in all fields— from science and inventions to the arts and social sciences—who had little or no formal academic education but were home tutored, allowed to experiment on their own, or were apprenticed to the trade of the profession they wished to follow.

In the twentieth century, one of the most outstanding examples of progress made by what I surmise were kinesthetic learning techniques employed naturally by employees is written about by Jon Gertner in *The Idea Factory: Bell Labs and the Great Age of American Innovation* (New York and London: Penguin Press, 2012).

The front inside dust jacket of his book sums up the core description that caught my attention. "From its beginnings in the 1920s until its demise in the 1980s, Bell Labs—officially, the research and development wing of AT&T—was the biggest, and arguably the best, laboratory for new ideas in the world. From the transistor to the laser, from digital communications to cellular telephony, it's hard to find an aspect of modern life that hasn't been touched by Bell Labs.

"At its heart, this is a story about the life and work of a small group of brilliant and eccentric men . . . who spent their careers at Bell Labs. Their job was to research and develop the future of communications. Small-town boys, childhood hobbyists, oddballs."

Listening to Gertner being interviewed on NPR (National Public Radio), I heard him speak of how the older inventors and scientists mentored the youngsters, opening the doors of experimentation and play so that the next big invention was born of hands-on learning by kinesthetic players. Speaking of apprenticeship learning, this was the last true hotbed of a method of learning and producing that the Western world has seen. Gone are the days when a person apprenticed with a doctor to become a doctor, or a person apprenticed with a lawyer to become a lawyer.

When Linear learning became the education of choice for the public school system, the only remaining kinesthetic learning took place at trade schools. There it produced a wide range of intelligent tradespeople who were often relegated to receive a lower wage than their academically trained peers and lower community status regardless of their level of intelligence.

Aside from these discrepancies, many young people attempting to further their education had to face entrance exams that had little to do with their major studies. And to exit their classes, they had to pass Linear tests with the "right" answers even if they could "show" that they had a thorough understanding of the material that was taught.

I would recommend that you first study in classes that reflect your passion. Your *True You* desires to see how you can learn what you need to learn in a kinesthetic way. Even if you don't get the best of grades, learn what you need to learn in order to reach your goals and produce the outcomes you desire and do it your way.

Words of Advice

Realize that you can learn any subject or body of professional material, no matter how complex, by utilizing kinesthetic learning with some support from Linear learning. Mari presented me with a clearly written example of what we're talking about now. As she was finishing the course she was taking in Microsoft Office, she sent me the following, having not only translated the way in which she needed to learn, but also how she began to teach others with predominant ADD skills to master the lessons, too. Here's her email response to my query about how school was going:

Here's a brief description of the challenges and accommodations I have found helpful.

Microsoft Office textbooks (Word, Excel, PowerPoint) are written in a very Linear fashion. Basically, you are given a very brief description of what is being done, and from there you are instructed to "hit" this key, then "hit" the next key, and so on and so forth, until the exercise is done.

I found this to be similar to being given directions by a GPS where you are told to "turn" here, proceed and then "turn" again at the next location. The problem is that without being able to visualize where I am headed, it is easy for me to become disoriented and confused.

What I had to do was review the entire chapter first and make notations at certain intervals. This way I was able to complete a "task" that then linked to the next "task" I would be performing which allowed the entire process to make sense for me. I have shared this with other students and it is working for us. Some of us just need the "Big Picture" clearly fixed in our minds before attempting new and unfamiliar tasks. An example would be traveling across country, which I have done alone several times. I map out (and make reservations) from the starting point to the midpoint (where I stop for the night), and then have another set of clear directions from the midpoint to the destination. It works every time!

What a beautifully stated accommodation to a Linear set of directions. Mari is definitely on her way to using her ADD brainstyle to advantage to be all she was meant to be.

An Inner Locus of Perception and Control and a Strong Sensing Capability

Our worldview comes from within ourselves and it both holds a steady projection within us of what and how we value, as well as providing an awareness that communicates with the outside world about what we see, feel, and in this case, sense.

Thus we are idiosyncratically guided from within ourselves rather than from outside. This perception allows us to hold a steady course based upon our belief system. As we learned in chapter 2 in relation to the Core Components of Human Nature, full maturity is not gained until we make our childhood values our own through the process of rethinking them in an adult context.

At that point of rethinking, we decide to either keep the same values with which we were raised or we take on a new belief that feels right to us. Therefore we shift from the expression of any action or thought because we *should* do it to an expression of the action because we *want* to do it. We have reached Self-Control only after we choose to do or not to do something because we have made the decision within ourselves as something we believe.

To apply this attribute to our project's organization and production, we must be totally honest with ourselves. The way our emotional system is made is such that if we do something that we truly don't want to do, but rather do it because we *should* do it, we have set ourselves up for failure. No matter how hard we work, it is likely that we will unconsciously sabotage the results. Sooner or later, we become our own worst enemy.

Do you tend to do what is expected of you or what an authority tells you is the *right* thing to do? (Not in a legal situation.) Briefly describe the situation:

_____

_____

Have you done something that you really didn't want to do but another part of you wanted to do it (such as helping a friend or family member)?

_____

_____

We know what to do by listening to our inner drumbeat, not by using a template produced outside of ourselves into which we are expected to fit. If you've tried to fit into something that wasn't a good *fit* for you, what happened?

_____

_____

If we take this a step further, if our project demands that we do something that is too hard, something that we have failed at before, perhaps multiple times, our psyche is not going to want to go down that path again. Has this happened to you? _____Briefly describe.

_____

_____

We've talked a lot about Chronic Stress Response (chapter 3). CSR is a perfect setup to induce failure. Obviously, each of us must watch out for this reaction so that we don't set ourselves up for a negative outcome. Do you have signs of Chronic Stress Response?)

_____ yes _____ no

If "yes", briefly describe the trigger(s) you face.

_____

_____

Do certain situations overwhelm your feelings or cause you a high level of anxiety?

_____ yes _____ no

If yes, briefly describe the situation(s). _____

_____

It's important to know that with your strong sensing capability, you have skills that others don't even know exist. You simply "know," since you have access to inner sensory visioning, inner experience, or intuition. You also may feel the sensing physically in your body. Once you've perceived an event on a sensory level, you can decide what to do in response. Have you had a situation where you felt a sensate response? _____ Describe what it was like.

_____

_____

What did you decide to do about what you felt?

_____

_____

You may even store information using this mechanism rather than by categorizing according to the labels in more general use. You may wish to practice being aware of externally invisible signs of sensate processing of information that comes to you by paying attention to what you sense, feel physically, emotionally, and even in picture form in your mind's eye.

I learned to edit by recognizing that I literally felt pressure inside my physical body. I noticed when something felt off with what I'd written. I have a particularly sensitive spot in my skull's right side about midway between the front and back of my head and an inch or two down from the top. I also have a small red light, about an inch in diameter that I see in my head midway between the front of my skull and back, only deeper toward the center—a light that goes on when I read something that's been miswritten.

I discovered the light when working with an editor who had already marked my work. Since I read to myself aloud in my head, I was able to discover the light before I actually saw her edit. I reasoned that if I picked up the sign ahead of time, then I could use it for the development of my own editing skills. And sure enough, as soon as I started to practice on my own by raising my conscious awareness of what I was seeing, feeling, and hearing, I began to edit pretty well.

I also became aware about forty years ago that I have what I call "feelings boxes" in my mind that are rectangular in shape. They house the records of feelings associated with previous experiences, not the cognitive information about the events. Turns out, I store information by feeling tones or the feelings themselves, not by dates, locations, names, and labels. I've tried explaining this to others, on occasion, but have not found out what is working here. But the cluster of events or happenings in any one box always belong together. These memories I don't forget. It's only my memory of labels and names that I struggle to remember.

All I can say is that it's my world. You'll need to pay attention and discover your world by utilizing your Analogue attributes. Listen as you proceed with projects and you'll be led by what is right to do (you'll feel it) and steer away from what makes you hesitant.

When you're working on your project your thinking mind will be functioning strategically. It's then that if you get an internal sensate feeling which is not cloaked in an emotional feeling tone, you'll know that your sensate capability is functioning. Practice will make perfect, or nearly so.

A High Level of Sensitivity: Sight, Sound, Taste, Smell, Touch, and Intuition

Our sensitivity (sometimes called "thin skin") is felt through our senses: sight, sound, taste, smell, and touch, as well as intuition. We often pick up cues that others don't experience. You may have certain sensitivities more developed than others. We're all different. For example, perhaps your vision is actually not too great and you don't pick up a lot of information that way. But your intuition is awesome and you can hear or touch something and know a whole lot more about the total situation than the person who has good eyes and stands in the same setting with you.

Being empathetic, that is, feeling what others are feeling, we often can provide support and caring to someone who is experiencing an intense emotional situation, whether happy or sad. It could be their joy at getting engaged to the person of their dreams, or it could be the sadness of watching their last child enter kindergarten on the way to growing up.

One of the signs of empathy is tearing up when you hear or see something emotional. We are responsive to our environments and can even pick up the tone of a room, a house, any space. In the writing of this book, I used three different libraries regularly and two additional ones on occasion. I can easily order them on a number of fronts. I can rank the libraries according to how the staff feels about their jobs. Same with grocery stores or any environment. I know if someone is having a good day or a bad day.

Some libraries have staff that loves to work with people and even the shy workers don't hold back with patrons. I would put my money on the management in that library. I'll bet the "boss" likes her or his job and shares the good feelings with each employee regularly. I'm sure they receive kudos and also have special times like on Fridays where they can all relax into the wearing of Texas jeans or have pastries brought in from the local bakery.

The head librarian probably likes most people, is sensitive to staff, and knows what to do to cultivate loyalty and trust. There's more smiling than grimaces. A good place to be!

Another library took a lot of work on my part to "break through" to individual staff. Everyone looked remorseful. Because I am so sensitive, I often make an effort to improve the mood of any place I have to be because otherwise I have to feel the "poor" feelings. It works and everyone wins.

Are you a sensitive person? If so, in what ways?

_____

_____

_____

Like me, many Analogue people can also be wounded when others do not see or sense the source of the wounding, yet we experience it nonetheless. Perhaps it's another's anger, sadness, or fear that we are picking up. And though we might have felt just fine ten minutes earlier, we may very quickly feel a lump in our throat or a stone in our heart. Are you very sensitive to other's emotions, catching the feeling by proximity to the person?

_____

_____

What is your reaction to being told you're too sensitive? Tell your story.

_____

_____

_____

_____

One of the best responses that it took me years to come up with when I was told, "You're too sensitive" was "I'm just the right amount sensitive for me." Ironically, it rarely happens anymore once I owned my sensitivity and didn't feel guilty or poorly when I was criticized. Of course, one of the reasons is that I don't hang out much with insensitive people. I can also spot a person from miles away that doesn't want to go anywhere near a sensitive or painful feeling. So I don't let my feeling out around that person. Problem solved.

Your Sensitivity is a skill that you need to both use and protect. It can open a door that leads into many an occupation and relationship. On the other hand, if you're not in an environment that *fits* you or you're with people and energy either at work or at home that is dysfunctional, harsh, thoughtless, and/or insensitive, you are likely to develop emotional symptoms.

Chronic Stress Response looks like there is something emotionally wrong with you when, in reality, your emotional system is trying to get your attention. You are or have been doing something(s), sometimes for a long time, that is bad for you or that doesn't *fit*. If you hadn't become angry or depressed, I'd wonder why.

Places to look for problems or frustrations in your life that affect your emotional sensitivity include current or historical experiences in your family or work settings.

Family Setting

There are family systems in which a behavior starts out as an innocent case of teasing, "Oh look at those chubby legs" or "Here comes 'air head.'" Such remarks used over a period of time wound subtly at first, but accumulate deeply over time. And they become abusive. When speakers are uncomfortable with their own feelings, and fail to own their inadequacies and discomforts, they may project their fears outward by using anger or criticism, veiled in "teasing." Hurtful damage is the result.

Other family members who don't put a stop to the comments are accomplices who are afraid the perpetrator may turn on them. They remain silent. And soon there is a need that only a family counselor trained in family dynamics can unwind, helping every-one to live supportively with one another.

Well-meaning family members who have not resolved their own pain and hurt carry their emotions with them. If you're a sensitive ADD person, you will likely be affected by these unintended and unattended emotions and experience them as if you'd caught an emotional cold.

There is also the major trauma insult to entire families when there is environmental or financial loss, loss of a family member, illness, or any of the many travesties that can befall us humans.

Job Setting

Verbal, physical, emotional, and sexual abuse from authorities, peers, clients, or customers can create chaos in your mind, anxiety, depression, and anger. Well-meaning colleagues and coworkers who have not resolved their own pain and hurt may be the source of "contamination" to your mood as you feel their pain. You're likely to know before most others if the business itself is in jeopardy or is being poorly run or skating outside of the law. You'll simply sense it. And you need to believe in yourself and act accordingly.

Consider the sources of positive energy and negative energy in your life. When you sum up the positives and negatives, you'll see your balance of stress and where it's coming from. Then you can consider what you can readily change, think about what you want to change and factor in more positives to balance life situations that you can't, or choose not to, change (such as a sick family member). It's amazing what an external support can do, such as a friend whom you see regularly—maybe someone you walk with every day or someone you play racquetball with once a week.

What you don't want to do is act on your sensitive antenna before you make sure you have the right to jump into a situation. If someone's life is in danger, of course, do what you must, though preferably call 911 rather than getting in the middle of a problem yourself.

But when you are "catching" the emotions of others and trying to rescue them, you sometimes may feel their emotions even more than they do. You could be setting yourself up to get into big trouble. It's better to either call for help or simply remove yourself from the situation and speak with a mutual friend or a stable person who knows the situation.

By simply being around people you may pick up another's rage or terror without realizing why you suddenly feel bad, out-of-control, or afraid.

If you suddenly become emotionally overwhelmed when you have been feeling fine a short time earlier, it's likely that you have come in contact with someone who has a serious emotional problem: rage, terror, depression. You don't have to know the person, but whether you do or you don't, remove yourself from the situation and recenter yourself, get grounded by walking, talking to someone whom you trust, do exercise, yoga, or some other physical activity.

Emotional Skill-Building to Help You Accommodate

In part because of the Sensitivity Attribute typical of an ADD brainstyle, it is important to recognize the ways in which expression of that sensitivity manifests through emotions and behavior, and also how you can learn to use it for protection, wisdom-building, and everyday functioning so you are able to reach and maintain your *True You* journey.

With most emotions, there is a good side and a bad side. Let's begin by looking at different sides of key emotional responses as they have to do with managing our style of brain construction.

Fear and doubt can show up as a response to being afraid of failure, of being embarrassed, of feeling helpless or hopeless when putting yourself out into the world. It may make starting a project or letting others see your work very hard to do. Fear that you will not live up to your dreams stifles your expression. Sadly, then no one knows you as you truly are.

To determine whether you ought to progress with an activity, you must decide whether there is a tangible block from your being able to achieve the outcome that is being asked of you. Or do you need to take small steps to get used to doing what you feel afraid of or doubtful about and keep working to overcome what has felt like a block so you can be true to yourself?

As you learned in chapter 2 about developing a Sense of Competence (p. 52), if you had your beginning self-esteem shaken by being abused or neglected early in your life, you may have lost confidence that you could achieve. When it came to trying something new, you would have been hesitant and fearful of making a mistake from then on.

To remedy that, you will need to take small steps with someone you trust who is not going to hurt you, or judge you, or push you. That means you'll have to trust the person.

Consider another scenario: Ask yourself whether you have had situations come up in which you felt fear and, indeed, it turns out something was amiss. Your job is to consider both experiences and progress forward slowly. Being sensitive, you need to study your feeling of fear to determine whether you need to listen to it or determine whether it would be to your advantage to "work through" it. In either case, you must not allow anyone to take total control of you so as to force you. Force always creates injury. You are not to be injured, but rather gentled into overcoming fear that you don't need to continue to carry.

Overcoming fears and doubts is important for a healthy, happy, productive life. You will find that as you learn more and more ways to accommodate your differences in brainstyle, as you move toward fulfilling your dream of living from your *True You*, the more you will want to gentle yourself into expanding your release of your fears and doubts.

Breathing is one of the most effective ways to reduce fear and actually train yourself to move through fear and doubt. Be cautious not to hyperventilate by gulping breath in order to try to take in more air. Even, moderate, regular breathing is in order.

Consider adding meditation to your breathing. Every time you exhale, picture letting the fear or doubts leave your mind and body. And with every breath you inhale, imagine that you are inhaling whatever you need: courage, strength, power, calm, peace, or whatever you feel will help you.

Body work such as massage, yoga, Tai chi, or any structured exercise you are drawn to that has breathing and control as a part of it will also help you to free yourself of fear and doubt.

Self-talk is a good idea. Tell your scared part whatever you feel that part needs to hear. If it's your inner child part, you may want to visualize yourself taking him or her by the hand and encouraging the child as you say, "I won't leave you. I once was scared but I've learned to have courage just as you are showing right now by doing _____. I'm really proud of you."

You don't need magical words. Just be real and talk from your heart. You'll learn from yourself.

There are many ways to overcome fear. Years ago when I was doing work in the television field, I was petrified of the station's chief. He had a huge amount of authority. He had a very Linear brainstyle . . . yes, I knew, even before I knew anything about ADD. He was quite authoritarian. What I knew was that I felt incredibly uncomfortable trying to communicate to him, and he didn't seem to resonate much to me. My "wrap someone around my finger charm" did absolutely no good with him. There sure wasn't trust or bonding between us. And in those days, I sure didn't have self-confidence to hold my own.

So I talked to a psychotherapist friend of mine and he suggested that I imagine in my mind's eye that the Chief was standing in front of me. I'm here to tell you I immediately began to perspire and get cold chills at the same time. Then I was to tell the Chief whatever it was that I wanted or needed to ask him, like, "Could I do a TV short about False Accusations?"

I couldn't think of anything else to say. My prompter said, "Okay, you're going to need to mentally shrink him down to the size of a child so you can tell him the value of your request." Well, yes, I could do that. As I did, I began to recall what I wanted to ask and I actually got the words out with my friend. I practiced a few more times and later in the day as I went to the station.

The first thing I did as I moved toward the Chief's desk was to visualize him the size of a child. My request not only came seamlessly out of my mouth, but it was granted and I made a three-and-a-half minute False Accusation tape for the following week that was well received.

I never again had as much trouble as that first time, no matter who I was confronting or greeting. Of course, as a therapist I had some helpful friends and we traded strengths. If you don't have that perk, then find a mentor or counselor who can do a one-time session with one of the forms of hypnosis or imagery and you'll likely gain a tool that will last you a lifetime.

Anxiety and nervousness can result from previous hurtful situations or can be hardwired biochemically. When we're talking about these responses in relation to ADD, I would ask you to think back about situations when you felt these ways.

If they seemed to appear in learning situations but not other places, I would suspect that you discovered very early that you could do some things that matched your level of intelligence while not being able to do what the majority of other kids could do who were no smarter.

The more nervous or anxious we become in certain situations may mean that we have the ability to understand or accomplish an outcome, but we need to do it in a way that is different from the way in which we are being asked to perform it. No matter how hard I tried to memorize things, I discovered early on that I had, and still have, very poor rote memory. Now ask me to tell a story or write a descriptive essay about almost any topic and you'll see that I have a solid, accurate sense of the subject. I can tell the tale. But I sure can't pass an exam that labels and defines every aspect by name.

Want to see anxious? Put me in a test situation, even the written part of a driving test. I can do the road test fine, but not the written part. I know what the road signs mean as I go down the highway and obey them, but ask me on a paper/digital test to tell you what the shape of the mileage sign is and I'm a goner.

Synchronicity! I had no sooner written this last paragraph than I received an email from Mari—yes, "our" Mari who has shared experiences of herself throughout the book. And Mari said: "Lynn. I just finished Microsoft PowerPoint (loved it!) and am now starting on Microsoft Outlook. I'm always a bit crazy when starting something new."

I can tell from her comment that the nervousness is there, but that it's not crippling, nor turning to depression and self-doubt. It's a great example of how we—as I suspect all human beings do—feel nervous when doing something that is new to us or that may or may not *fit* our brainstyle. But we trudge forward knowing that we probably have a pretty good chance of making good. "Kudos, Mari, you have just the right amount of nervousness for starting something new."

My suggestion to you is to not judge yourself, your worth, skill level, or intelligence by the way in which society generally measures such things. Read your own reactions to the situations, that is, anxiety or doubt levels, and pick and choose the way you wish to proceed with your life. It's okay to be selfish and discriminating.

If you have a certifiable anxiety disorder or traumatic nervous response, *please do* get professional help. Check with your primary care physician or a mental health professional and get the help you deserve. If you've been subjected to serious trauma and loss in the recent past, get the support you need from the professionals who know how to properly monitor medication.

And, *just* because you are both ADD and have a major stress reaction, remember, they are not comorbid—because your brainstyle is *not* a disease. You are a person with an Analogue brainstyle who happens to have had some hard times and you deserve to feel better. Hopefully you'll find someone who is sufficiently knowledgeable about ADD to honor your brainstyle and build you up, mending your life so that you can meet up with your *True You* as you heal.

Last but not least, though hesitation and anticipation are totally different from one another, they accomplish the same task for us. Because they measure how we feel about undertaking or continuing something, they serve to guide our behavior with regard to moving into action.

The general rule of thumb is to hesitate about doing whatever you're considering if you feel hesitation. And if you feel anticipation, you're probably on the right track to continue with your choice to act.

If you're dealing with hesitation about wanting to buy a special object, the hesitation doesn't mean you absolutely ought to give up on what you're considering. It may be a matter of timing. Perhaps you don't have the reserves to spend money at this time. Maybe later. Perhaps you need to do more shopping first. Or maybe your birthday is coming up and several people know you want this object. The hesitation is attached to this time and situation. Listen, Watch, and then Decide.

Let's say that you felt anticipation about going on a trip, but the one that you had decided upon was cancelled. Now you're not sure whether another one could replace the cancelled one. You don't want to be disappointed. The Travel Agent asked you to go by the agency on your lunch hour and she'd have four or five alternative trip information packets available for you to consider.

You start to feel torn: should you go? What if you don't feel as good about one of the new ones as you did about the cancelled one? Maybe you should avoid the whole thing. Oh, you think, "What should I do?"

In this situation, all you have to remember to do is pay attention to your feelings of hesitation or anticipation as you look at the packets. Trust how you feel and you'll end up okay.

If the new ones don't make your heart beat faster, then forget about taking a trip for now. Remember, now is not forever.

However, you might find that as the agent is showing you the alternative trip packages, you see one you've not thought of before and it makes you feel excited. You find yourself figuring out the dates in relation to the time you can take off. You wonder about number of stops at key ports. You are eager to learn everything you can about the trip. You feel anticipation and want to go.

There's your answer! Enjoy.

HOW NICE TO HAVE LEARNED HOW TO PROTECT THE *TRUE YOU*: A WORK IN PROGRESS

Accommodation is the gift of protection for the evolved *True You* that you've been finding and building throughout this book. You've come so very, very far.

You've forgiven the earlier evolutions of the Wounded You who were unable to self-protect the wonderful person you were harboring within but had not yet been able to experience for yourself. You've found ways to heal so that you became ready to let the *True You* loose into the Linear culture of the modern age. And you've made choices based on the wisdoms passed down to you by those who have gone before so that you could appreciate the brainstyle that works for you.

You discovered that you had multiple Analogue Attributes that have ended up serving you magnificently. Part of the discovery has been that you can do anything anyone who is not ADD can do. You simply have to do it in your own way. And now you can recognize what those ways are, and I promise you, they don't take the genius of a rocket scientist. They only take the genius of *You*.

Remember to listen to the Self-Gratitude that your progress has been providing for you. Do you hear it now? Such gratitude for:

- Organizing using the Popcorn Popping Method
- Sorting out the pros and cons of having a high activity level: physically, mentally, emotionally, and verbally
- Following the model provided to support the development of Bell Lab's Idea Factory, where kinesthetic performing engineers, scientists, and laboratory workers performed brilliantly
- Housecleaning the debris left by fears, self-doubt, guilt, and low self-esteem guided by your Inner Locus of Control
- Learning to follow Mari's example of translating Linear teaching guidelines into Analogue Processing guidelines for you to get the Big Picture
- Overcoming the downside of ADD Sensitivity by building an armory of Accommodation Skills for the *True You* to use
- Becoming a master reader of your feelings so that they will guide you, teach you, and make you whole so that the end result will be a tool you can Trust in your own best interest, and
- Developing the Accommodating You to walk hand in hand with the *True You* and the Wounded You: a Triumvirate of Greatness.

EPILOGUE

TO MY READERS

This book has been a book about you and me and many others who have shared their stories so we could learn the truth about ourselves—a truth that is of great value to all with whom we live and come in contact, as well as a truth that is dedicated to our own good. It is a truth to be shared with those we love and those we will meet as we live out the rest of our lives.

By changing our perspective on the particular, wonderful style of brain construction with which we were born, we have had the opportunity to change an errant belief in our culture about the definition and value of how we experience, associate, and express everything we do.

Labeled as deficient and disordered, we have had the opportunity to see that neither of these definitions is true. Instead, we have been given the opportunity to see ourselves as simply different from some others of our kin. We have been given the freeing concept of diversity to embrace a judgment-free definition of ourselves. And, in so doing, we have become free to be who we are intended to be.

Throughout this book, we have had the chance to see the Analogue and Linear Attributes that we carry and that swirl around us from the culture in which we live. Hopefully, we can now distinguish between those attributes that are taught to us as *shoulds*—how we *should* experience, adapt, and act as defined by the majority culture—and the ways in which we are organically and naturally made that are equally of value.

If you would like to continue this conversation, please feel free to reach out to our community on my website: www.LynnWeiss. com. You will always be welcome there.

Lynn Weiss, PhD